FIND YOUR FOOD TRIGGERS

Investigate Every Food. Explore Low Lectin, Low Histamine, Low Oxalate, Low Salicylate Diets, DASH Diet, Diverticulitis Diet and Lots More.

BY THE FOOD HEROES

Copyright: The Food Heroes 2022. All rights reserved. No part of this guide may be reproduced in any form without permission in writing from the publisher except with brief quotations embodied in critical articles or reviews.

LEGAL & DISCLAIMER

The information in this book is not designed to replace or take the place of any form of medicine or professional medical advice. The information in this book has been provided for educational and entertainment purposes only.

You need to consult a professional medical practitioner in order to ensure you are both healthy enough and able to make use of this information. Always consult your professional medical practitioner before undertaking any new dietary regime, and particularly after reading this book.

The information in this book has been compiled from sources deemed reliable, and it is accurate to the best of the Author's knowledge; however, the Author cannot guarantee its accuracy and validity and cannot be held liable for any errors or omissions.

You must consult your doctor or get professional medical advice before using any suggested information in this book. This guide is not suitable for allergies.

While every care has been made to ensure accurate information, The Food Heroes accept no liability or responsibility for any errors or omissions. Always read product labels and do not rely solely on this information.

Upon using the information in this book, you agree to hold harmless the Author, and Publisher, from and against any damages, costs, and expenses, including any legal fees potentially resulting from the application of the information provided by this guide. This disclaimer applies to any damages or injury caused by the use and application, whether directly or indirectly, of any advice or information presented, whether for breach of contract, tort, negligence, personal injury, criminal intent, or under any other cause of action. You agree to accept all risks of using the information presented inside this book.

CONTENTS

INTRODUCTION 11
HOW TO USE 13
FIND YOUR FOOD TRIGGERS A-Z 15
    Acerola 15
    Agave syrup 15
    Alcohol 16
    Algae 17
    Almond 17
    Anchovies 18
    Apple 19
    Apple cider vinegar (ACV) 19
    Apricot 20
    Artichokes 20
    Artificial sweeteners 21
    Asparagus 21
    Aubergine 22
    Avocado 22
    Bamboo shoots 23
    Banana 23
    Barley 24
    Barley malt, malt 24
    Basil 25
    Beans 25
    Beef 26
    Beer 26
    Beetroot 27
    Bell pepper (hot or sweet) 28
    Bison 28
    Bivalves (mussels, oysters, clams, scallops) 29
    Black caraway 29
    Blackberry 30
    Blackcurrants 30
    Blue cheeses 31
    Blue fenugreek 31
    Blueberries 32
    Bok choi 32
    Borlotti beans 33
    Bouillon 33

- Boysenberry 34
- Brandy 34
- Brazil nut 35
- Bread 35
- Broad-leaved garlic 36
- Broad beans 37
- Broccoli 37
- Brussels sprouts 38
- Buckwheat 38
- Butter 38
- Cabbage 39
- Cactus pear 40
- Cardamom 40
- Carrot 41
- Cashew nut 41
- Cassava 42
- Cauliflower 42
- Celery 43
- Cep mushrooms 43
- Chamomile and chamomile tea 44
- Champagne 44
- Chard 45
- Cheddar cheese 45
- Cheese made from unpasteurized "raw" milk 46
- Cheeses 46
- Cherry 47
- Chia, chia seeds 48
- Chicken 48
- Chickpeas 49
- Chicory 49
- Chili pepper, red, fresh 50
- Chives 50
- Chocolate 51
- Cilantro 52
- Cinnamon 52
- Citrus fruits 53
- Clover 53
- Cloves 54
- Cocoa butter and cacao butter 54
- Cocoa drinks, powder, etc 55
- Coconut and coconut derivatives 55
- Coffee 56
- Coriander 57
- Cornflakes 57
- Courgette 57
- Crab 58
- Cranberries and cranberry juice 58
- Crawfish 59
- Crayfish 59
- Cream cheeses 60

Cream	60
Cress	61
Cucumber	61
Cumin	62
Curry	62
Dates	63
Dextrose	64
Dill	64
Dragon fruit	64
Dried fruit	65
Dried meat	66
Dry-cured meats	66
Duck	67
Egg white	67
Egg yolk	68
Elderflower cordial	68
Endive	69
Espresso	69
Fennel	70
Fenugreek	70
Feta cheese	70
Figs (fresh or dried)	71
Fish	72
Flaxseed (linseed)	72
Fructose (fruit sugar)	73
Game (meat)	73
Garlic	74
Ginger	74
Goat's milk	75
Goji berry	75
Goose (organic, freshly cooked)	76
Gooseberry, gooseberries	76
Gouda cheese	77
Grapefruit	77
Grapes	78
Green beans	78
Green peas	79
Green tea	79
Guava	80
Ham (dried, cured)	80
Hazelnut	81
Hemp seeds (Cannabis sativa)	81
Herbal tea	82
Honey	82
Horseradish	83
Juniper berries	83
Kale	84
Kefir	84
Kelp	85
Kiwi	85

- Kohlrabi 86
- Lamb 86
- Lamb's lettuce, corn salad 87
- Lard 87
- Leek 88
- Lemon 88
- Lentils 88
- Lettuce 89
- Lime 89
- Liquor 90
- Liquorice 90
- Lobster 91
- Loganberry 91
- Lychee 92
- Macadamia 92
- Malt 93
- Malt extract 93
- Maltodextrin 94
- Mandarin orange 94
- Mango 95
- Maple syrup 95
- Margarine 95
- Marrow 96
- Mascarpone cheese 96
- Mate tea 97
- Melon 98
- Milk 98
- Millet 99
- Minced meat 99
- Mint 100
- Morel 100
- Morello cherries 101
- Mozzarella cheese 101
- Mulberry 102
- Mung beans (germinated, sprouting) 102
- Mushrooms, different types 103
- Mustard and mustard seeds 103
- Napa cabbage 103
- Nectarine 104
- Nettle tea 104
- Nori seaweed 105
- Nutmeg 106
- Nuts (see individual nuts for more details) 106
- Oats 107
- Olive oil 107
- Olives 108
- Onion 108
- Orange 109
- Oregano 109
- Ostrich 110

Oyster	110
Papaya	111
Parsley	111
Parsnip	112
Passionfruit	112
Pasta	113
Peach	113
Peanuts	114
Pear	114
Peas (green)	115
Pea Shoots (or pea sprouts)	115
Peppermint tea	116
Pickled food	116
Pineapple	117
Pistachio	117
Plum	118
Pomegranate	118
Poppy seeds	119
Pork	119
Potato	119
Poultry meat	120
Prawn	121
Processed cheese	121
Prune	122
Pulses	122
Pumpkin seed oil	123
Pumpkin	123
Pumpkin seeds	124
Quinoa	124
Rabbit	124
Raclette cheese	125
Radish	125
Raisins	126
Rapeseed oil (called canola oil in the US)	126
Raspberry	127
Red cabbage	127
Red wine vinegar	128
Redcurrants	128
Rhubarb	129
Rice	129
Rice cakes	130
Rice milk	130
Rice noodles	131
Ricotta cheese	131
Rooibos tea	132
Roquefort cheese	132
Rosemary	133
Rum	133
Rye	134
Sage	134

Salami	134
Salmon	135
Sauerkraut	135
Sausages of all kinds	136
Savoy cabbage	136
Schnapps	137
Seafood	137
Seaweed	138
Sesame	138
Sheep's milk, sheep milk	139
Shellfish	139
Shrimp	140
Smoked fish	140
Smoked meat	140
Snow peas	141
Soft cheese	141
Sour cream	142
Soy (soybeans, soy flour)	143
Soy sauce	143
Sparkling wine	144
Spelt	144
Spinach	145
Spirits	145
Squashes	146
Stevia	146
Stinging nettle	147
Strawberry	147
Sugar	148
Sunflower oil	148
Sunflower seeds	149
Sweetcorn	149
Sweet potato	150
Tea, black	150
Thyme	151
Tomato	151
Trout	152
Tuna	152
Turkey	153
Turmeric	153
Turnip	154
Vanilla	154
Venison	155
Vinegar: balsamic	155
Vinegar: distilled white vinegar	156
Walnut	156
Watercress	156
Watermelon	157
Wheat	157
Wheat germ	158
White button mushroom	158

Contents

Wild rice 159
Wine 159
Yam 160
Yeast 161
Yogurt/Yoghurt 161
Zucchini 162

SOURCES 163

INTRODUCTION

Food issues, intolerances and triggers are becoming more common all the time. They currently affect 15-20% of the population (source: *Medical News Today*). It now isn't unusual to have multiple food triggers, and clearly, people are finding it tougher than ever to figure out what exactly is causing the issues.

Enter *Find Your Food Triggers*.

We wanted to create one comprehensive guide to help you find those difficult foods that have been causing you major problems.

By 'triggers' we mean any food that causes negative symptoms and issues such as; IBS, digestion issues, hives, migraines, hypertension, fatigue and so on.

This guide is all about helping you navigate the world of complex diets. We wrote it because we have multiple food triggers ourselves. Yep, we're sensitive.

It frustrated us at how so much information out there seems to confuse us and conflict with other sources. Often, one list will tell you food is a trigger, and another will disagree. That's not helpful. In this guide, we have studied the best information and brought it together in one place.

So what is your food trigger? It's easy to find out, and then stay on top of your chosen diet.

Step 1: Look up any food/drink in our Find Your Food Triggers A-Z
Step 2: Check it against the following food triggers:

- **Diverticulitis**: Diverticulitis is a condition that affects the digestive tract. Diverticulitis and Diverticulosis are common in older adults, and doctors usually recommend a 3-stage diet.
- **Histamine**: The ever-increasing amount of histamine intolerance sufferers have a frustratingly wide range of symptoms. It's really tough to 'know every food' in terms of histamine levels (which is where we come in).
- **Hypertension**: You'll see references to the DASH Diet throughout. This stands for *Dietary Approaches to Stop Hypertension*. This limits sodium, saturated fat and added sugars and favors nutrients that help control blood pressure.
- **Lectins**: The Low-Lectin Diet is hugely popular and has helped millions. Eliminating lectins can help with digestive issues and inflammation, but it's tough to remember which foods are high in lectins. Our A-Z does it for you.
- **Oxalates**: When some people eat high-oxalate foods, the oxalates build up and their bodies can't get rid of it. Significant numbers of people benefit from eating a low-oxalate diet, and you can follow it here.
- **Salicylates**: Salicylates can cause adverse reactions to those who are sensitive, with a long list of symptoms. The key is to limit the side effects by avoiding high salicylate foods (listed here).

Many suffer from a combination of issues. For example, people who are histamine intolerant are often triggered by lectins too. That's one of the reasons this guide is so helpful. You can look up one food, and at a glance check all the different potential triggers. In addition, you may be searching for triggers, or you may already be following a particular diet already.

Now for a note on allergies: After careful consideration we have not listed the 14 principle allergens in this guide (for example, gluten, dairy, shellfish). That's because this guide is about finding triggers and intolerances, and allergies are a different category. As always though, consult your doctor before starting any new diet or regime.

We believe our list is the most comprehensive out there, and where there is debate, we have deferred to our top sources listed in the index at the back of the book.

With all that said, there will be areas you disagree on and that is why a) approach any potential trigger with caution, and b) always consult your medical practitioner before making any dietary changes. We know this list will never be definitive, and we pledge to continue to refine it as more information becomes available.

It's also important to point out that not everybody is triggered by certain foods. Not everybody needs to follow the listed diets in this book, nor wants to. All of which means you should consult with your practitioner to determine the correct course for you. Please keep in mind that materials and resources like this book are no substitute for medical advice and not intended as such.

We are a team of health writers who have researched food triggers in-depth. There's a lot of conflicting information out there and trust us, we feel your frustration. That's why we wanted to compile a comprehensive guide that's easy to understand so you can navigate your food triggers and heal.

HOW TO USE THE FIND YOUR FOOD TRIGGERS A-Z

This book works like a dictionary. Look for a food, drink or ingredient alphabetically or on search. We've introduced an emoji-based system based on careful analysis of the world's best sources to help you identify food triggers.

✓ = less likely to be a trigger
😐 = opinion is split, or not enough information
✗ = more likely to be a trigger

So, for example, on a low-lectin diet, you would look to eat more ✓ foods and cut out more ✗ (trigger) foods.

Respected sites often disagree on major foods. We reflect this where possible, but always work with your practitioner on determining the best foods for you.

DASH (Hypertension) notes

For the DASH diet, you'll find the following nutritional values per 100 grams based on the USDA database (unless stated otherwise);

- Saturated fat content
- Sodium content
- Sugar content

To avoid triggers on this diet, you'll want to aim for:

- One gram or less per serving of saturated fat
- Foods less than five percent of the daily value of sodium and less than 140 mg of sodium per serving
- Less than five grams of sugar per 100g

(sources: *NIH, FDA, NHS*)

Diverticulitis notes

There tend to be three stages to the 'Diverticulitis Diet'. If you suspect food triggers for Diverticulitis, your doctor will advise you on which stage to follow, depending on the severity of your symptoms.

- Stage One — Clear Liquids Diet. When you have diverticulitis, it's important to give your digestive system a break. That's why your doctor may have advised Stage One for at least three to five days.
- Stage Two — Low-Fiber Diet. You can slowly start adding low-fiber foods back into your diet.
- Stage Three — High-Fiber Diet. The maintenance stage. You can slowly add higher-fiber foods back into your diet to prevent having to go back to Stage One and Stage Two.

Disclaimer. You must consult your doctor or get professional medical advice before using any suggested information in this book.

This book is for informational purposes only. Always consult your health professional before changing your regime.

This book has been a labor of love, but it has been a challenge to put together as the major lists often disagree on the best approach for individual foods. We take no responsibility for our sources providing information that may not reflect your own experience.

So this is a guide, not a definitive list. Everybody is individual. That means we may list a food as being suitable for most people, but it will not be suitable for you. That is the nature of food triggers and intolerances and why it's so helpful to have guides like this, but you must consult your practitioner before using this book.

FOOD GUIDE

Acerola
- DASH: Fat: ✓ Sodium: ✓ Sugar: ✗
- Diverticulitis: Stage 1: ✗ Stage 2: ✓ Stage 3: ✓
- Histamine: ✓
- Lectin: 😐
- Oxalate: 😐
- Salicylates: ✗

Also known as *Barbados Cherries*. A fruit similar to a cherry, also red when it's ripe. Acerola is a rich source of vitamin C and contains many minerals and other vitamins like beta-carotene.

DASH Diet (Hypertension) (Hypertension): Acerola is low in saturated fat and sodium content however, acerola juice is high in sugar so avoid juicing this fruit. *Saturated fat content: 0.1g (per 100g), Sodium content: 7mg (per 100g) less than 1% daily value based on a 2,000 calorie diet, Sugar content: Not reported by the USDA however, a 1-cup serving of raw acerola juice contains 11g of sugar (source: Livestrong).*

Diverticulitis: No solid foods can be eaten at stage one, the clear liquids diet.

Histamine: Cherries tend to be lower histamine but there is sometimes some debate.

Lectins: Having scoured the research we have found only limited information. Given that acerola is like cherries, it may be low in lectins.

Oxalates: In large doses, it might cause kidney stones in some people.

Salicylates: There isn't much information available on the amount of salicylates acerola specifically contains (welcome to the frustrations of salicylate issues). The *Go Figure* website notes acerola may cause salicylate issues in sensitive individuals. We believe as cherries contain a high content, it's best to avoid or limit them.

Agave syrup
- DASH: Fat: ✓ Sodium: ✓ Sugar: ✗
- Diverticulitis: Stage 1: ✓ Stage 2: ✓ Stage 3: ✗
- Histamine: ✓
- Lectin: ✗
- Oxalate: 😐
- Salicylates: 😐

Also known as *agave nectar*.

DASH Diet (Hypertension): Low in sodium and saturated fat but thought to be high in sugar content. Avoid. *Saturated fat content: 0g (per 100g), Sodium content: 4mg (per 100g), less than 1% daily value based on a 2,000 calorie diet, Sugar content: 68g (per 100g).*

Diverticulitis: Agave syrup is clear so it is allowed at stage one, clear liquid diet. Also allowed at stage two, low-fiber diet.

Histamine: Eat in moderation. A lower sugar diet is generally healthier. This also applies to agave nectar.

Lectins: Agave itself and agave syrup are thought to be high in lectins.

Oxalates: One of those very confusing ingredients that is listed as low oxalate on many lists, but agave itself is listed as very high on many other lists. Therefore we wanted to write this book, and ultimately, if you want to eat agave on a low-oxalate diet, proceed with great caution as there is some debate about the oxalate content.

Salicylates: While honey and most sweets tend to be high in salicylates, agave syrup are thought to contain a more moderate amount. The way that it is processed - using heat and enzymes - destroys health-promoting benefits from the agave plant. Limit your use and proceed with caution.

Alcohol

- DASH: Fat: ✔ Sodium: ✔ Sugar: ✔
- Diverticulitis: Stage 1: ✘ Stage 2: ✘ Stage 3: ✘
- Histamine: ✘
- Lectin: 🤔
- Oxalate: ✔
- Salicylates: ✘

DASH Diet (Hypertension): Alcohol is low in saturated fat, sodium and sugar content. The sugar content will vary depending on the type of alcohol so we recommend you check the nutritional values for each drink carefully. Healthline recommends drinking alcohol sparingly on the DASH diet. You don't have to eliminate alcohol completely although it's good to limit consumption. PubMed have published a study concluding: *"A high DASH score and a reduction in alcohol consumption could be effective nutritional strategies to prevent hypertension."* Another study by the U.S. Department of Veterans Affairs found: *"Participants who increased their alcohol intake also increased their rate of unhealthy eating." Saturated fat content: 0g (per 100g), Sodium content: 4mg (per 100g) less than 1% daily value based on a 2,000 calorie diet, Sugar content: 0g (per 100g).*

Diverticulitis: The general rule is to avoid alcohol, but the science is mixed. Alcohol is seen as a risk factor for several gastrointestinal issues. There are many who cannot tolerate alcohol, although there are some who seem to manage some alcoholic beverages as part of their daily diet. The key is finding the right balance.

Histamine: Alcohols are some of the most problematic things you can drink on a low histamine diet. The Healing Histamine Site notes that alcohol itself isn't always high histamine but has the effect of blocking DAO (diamine oxidase) production. The prospect of giving up alcohol often comes as a bit of a shock to people starting a histamine diet for the first time. Don't be disheartened if you are new to this. Start by cutting out alcohol and once you reduce your histamine levels re-introduce slowly. Wines are often extremely problematic although some low-histamine wines can be found. But note the DAO-blocking element above. Alcohols contain histamine-degrading enzymes, but some rums, tequilas and Tito's Vodka may be purer than others. We have seen some claims online that plain vodka, gin and white rum are all low in histamine - these may be better options than other alcohols, but they still may block your DAO enzyme and therefore cause a histamine reaction.

Lectins: Content varies so check individual alcohols for further detail. Beer should be avoided as it's thought to be high in lectins. Red wine contains high levels of Polyphenols (antioxidants) compared to other types of wine (including white wine) however, it's thought to also contain lectins. Some experts allow drinking wine high in Polyphenols (in moderation) on a low-lectin diet. Test red wine carefully. It's unclear whether sparkling wine, brandy, rum, spirits and schnapps should be avoided. Drink in moderation and test carefully. Dessert wines, sweet wines and white wines should also be avoided. Given the high sugar content, these wines also don't seem to have the same benefits as red wine. Tequila is something that many seem to enjoy on a low-lectin diet, but again, test carefully.

Oxalates: Beer is thought to be low-oxalate. Red wine and white wine are thought to be very low, and liquor extremely low. So alcohol actually gets a good emoji in our list. With of course, the usual caveats about other health-related issues linked to alcohol. Alcohol might often be low oxalate, but it might also not be good for your health.

Salicylates: Alcoholic beverages like beer, wine, and spirits such as rum and sherry contain a high level of salicylates. Champagne and sparkling wine are on the higher end, with Drambuie containing one of the highest levels for a liqueur. Dry white wines have a lower amount while beer and ale can range anywhere from .32 to 1.26 per 100 g. Of course, there are also negative health effects of alcohol to consider.

Algae
- DASH: Fat: ✗ Sodium: ✗ Sugar: ✓
- Diverticulitis: Stage 1: ✗ Stage 2: ✗ Stage 3: ✓
- Histamine: ✗
- Lectin: ✓
- Oxalate: ✓
- Salicylates: 🤐

DASH Diet (Hypertension): Low in sugar but thought to be high in saturated fat and sodium content. Avoid. *Saturated fat content: 2g (per 100g), Sodium content: 812mg (per 100g) 35% daily value based on a 2,000 calorie diet, Sugar content: 3.07g (per 100g)* (source: *Fatsecret Platform API*).

Diverticulitis: No solid foods can be eaten at stage one, the clear liquids diet. It's thought that red algae and brown algae have high levels of fiber content so allowed at the high-fiber stage.

Histamine: Several supplements contain algae and we have found these to cause a reaction too.

Lectins: Thought to be low in lectins. Red algae should be avoided as these are high in lectins and often consumed raw.

Oxalates: Related to Algae, phycocyanin in spirulina (a blue-green algae) can protect cells from oxalates. This is according to a research article published by the National Institute of Health.

Salicylates: There isn't a lot of information available related to salicylates and algae. However, spirulina, a blue-green algae known for its many health benefits has been well-documented in studies to contain an active compound called C-phycocyanin. This component was shown to significantly reduce tinnitus secondary to high amounts of salicylates which may show that it is a low salicylate food. This is not conclusive though; proceed with caution.

Almond
- DASH: Fat: ✗ Sodium: ✓ Sugar: ✓
- Diverticulitis: Stage 1: ✗ Stage 2: ✗ Stage 3: ✓
- Histamine: 🤐
- Lectin: 🤐
- Oxalate: ✗
- Salicylates: ✗

DASH Diet (Hypertension): Almonds may be enjoyed as part of a healthy diet as long as you eat only 4-5 servings a week. Eating Well's website notes almonds as part of the DASH diet and a heart-healthy lifestyle. PubMed have published a study concluding: *"Almonds might have a considerable favorite effect in blood pressure and especially in diastolic blood pressure, and it could be encouraged as part of a healthy diet; however, because of the high calorie content, the intake should be part of a healthy diet."* Saturated fat content: 3.8g (per 100g), Sodium content: 1mg (per 100g) less than 1% daily value based on a 2,000 calorie diet, Sugar content: 4.35g (per 100g).

Diverticulitis: No solid foods can be eaten at stage one, the clear liquids diet. Almonds are high in fiber.

Histamine: According to Mast Cell 360, small amounts are well tolerated. This is one of those foods that we have found we tolerate intermittently. Sometimes they cause a reaction but tend to be fine in very small doses. As always with histamine intolerance, everybody is different. Test in very small quantities initially.

Lectins: Almond skin is high in lectins. Here is a top tip to enjoy almonds: you can eat lower-lectin almonds by removing the skin and blanching them to lower the lectin content. Soaking and blanching will be your friend for living with lectin sensitivities.

Oxalates: With almonds, and all nuts, there is an issue with portion control. One or two almonds will probably be okay for you. However, the whole packet = lots of oxalates. Almonds can quickly cause oxalate issues. Some say all nuts should be avoided on a Low-Oxalate diet. Almonds and Brazil nuts are thought to be high. According to the University of Chicago, almonds contain 122mg per serving.

Salicylates: Almonds are thought to contain a high level of salicylates.
They do have other health benefits - they aid in the regeneration of the nervous system and have many other benefits. They are a good supply of protein and iron, and beneficial for vegans and vegetarians; however, when limiting salicylates, it's best to eat a small amount, just one to three rather than a handful.

Anchovies

- DASH: Fat: ✗ Sodium: ✗ Sugar: ✓
- Diverticulitis: Stage 1: ✗ Stage 2: ✓ Stage 3: ✗
- Histamine: ✗
- Lectin: ✓
- Oxalate: ✓
- Salicylates: ✓

Top tip: if anchovies are allowed on the diet, opt for wild caught anchovies as these are supposed to contain higher levels of omega-3s.

DASH Diet (Hypertension): Low in sugar but thought to be high in saturated fat and sodium content. Avoid. *Saturated fat content: 2.2g (per 100g), Sodium content: 3,668 mg (per 100g), 152% daily value based on a 2,000 calorie diet, Sugar content: 0g (per 100g).*

Diverticulitis: No solid foods can be eaten at stage one, the clear liquids diet. Anchovies contain no fiber so they're allowed on the low-fiber diet.

Histamine: Most fish are very high in histamine. Ideally fish should be frozen within one hour of catching, and even then anchovies are poorly tolerated. Other fish may be better.

Lectin: Low in lectins.

Oxalates: Low in oxalates, but thought to be high in purines, which also cause kidney stones – uric ones, not calcium oxalate, which are the most common kind.

Salicylates: Anchovies are considered to be low in salicylates and rich in omega-3 fatty acids which offer powerful benefits for heart health, including reducing blood pressure and triglyceride levels. They also contain a high level of B3 and selenium.

Apple

- DASH: Fat: ✓ Sodium: ✓ Sugar: ✗
- Diverticulitis: Stage 1: ✗ Stage 2: 😷 Stage 3: ✓
- Histamine: ✓
- Lectin: ✓
- Oxalate: ✓
- Salicylates: ✗

Note the high sugar content in apples. According to the US Department of Agriculture, a medium-sized apple contains approximately 19g of sugar.

DASH Diet (Hypertension): Eat in moderation. *Saturated fat content: 0g (per 100g), Sodium content: 1mg (per 100g), less than 1% daily value based on a 2,000 calorie diet, Sugar content: 10g (per 100g).*

Diverticulitis: No solid foods can be eaten at stage one, the clear liquids diet. At stage two, the low-fiber diet, peel and deseed the apple. Test carefully.

Histamine: Apples are thought to potentially lower your histamine levels.

Lectins: Low in lectins. Best to eat when the apple is in season. It's thought that fruits in season may contain fewer lectins than when they're out of season.

Oxalates*:* Thought to be low oxalate.

Salicylates*:* Salicylate content can vary wildly with apples, so it is worth proceeding with caution. The amount of salicylates in apples is thought to depend on the type of apple. And people wonder why salicylate intolerance is confusing!   Golden and Red Delicious are thought to contain the least at .1-.25 milligrams (mg) per 100 grams (g), while Granny Smith have the highest level at .5 – 1 mg. Be aware that some sources, including WebMD, recommend avoiding apples altogether so proceed carefully.

Apple cider vinegar (ACV)

- DASH: Fat: ✓ Sodium: ✓ Sugar: ✓
- Diverticulitis: Stage 1: ✗ Stage 2: ✓ Stage 3: ✗
- Histamine: 😷
- Lectin: ✓
- Oxalate: ✓
- Salicylates: 😷

DASH Diet (Hypertension): Allowed on the DASH diet. Studies have shown apple cider vinegar to lower post-meal blood glucose (source: *The University of Chicago Medical Center*). *Saturated fat content: 0g (per 100g), Sodium content: 5mg (per 100g), less than 1% daily value based on a 2,000 calorie diet, Sugar content: 0.4g (per 100g).*

Diverticulitis: Allowed on the low-fiber diet.

Histamine: The best-tolerated vinegar. Many find this acceptable, but still, many do not. If it doesn't suit you, search for 'verjus' which many in the low-histamine world love. It works similarly to ACV but is low in histamine.

Lectins: It's thought that all types of vinegar are acceptable on a low-lectin diet. To decrease lectin content in foods, *"adding a tiny splash of apple cider vinegar to soak water may help neutralize the lectins further"* (source: *Simply Nourished Nutrition*).

Oxalates: Low oxalate. The website Healthline notes an additional benefit.
Some people recommend using ACV as a natural way to treat kidney stones. The acetic acid found in ACV is thought to soften, break down, and dissolve kidney stones. Kidney stones can be reduced in size so that you can easily pass them in your urine.

Salicylates: Opinion is split. ACV in foods may not cause a problem; however, taking it as a supplement and/or drinking it straight is not advised because of the high level of salicylates. The website Allergenics notes; "*Sauces and Condiments: most commercial or store-bought gravies, sauces and pastes (e.g. tomato paste, Worcester sauce, gravy mix), jams, marmalades, fruit/mint/honey flavoring, chewing gum, white and cider vinegars*".

Apricot

- DASH: Fat: ✓ Sodium: ✓ Sugar: ✗
- Diverticulitis: Stage 1: ✗ Stage 2: 😐 Stage 3: ✓
- Histamine: ✓
- Lectin: ✓
- Oxalate: ✓
- Salicylates: ✗

DASH Diet (Hypertension): Low in saturated fat and sodium content but high in sugar. Eat in moderation. *Saturated fat content: 0g (per 100g), Sodium content: 1mg (per 100g) less than 1% daily value based on a 2,000 calorie diet, Sugar content: 9g (per 100g).*

Diverticulitis: No solid foods can be eaten at stage one, the clear liquids diet. At stage two, the low-fiber diet, peel and deseed the apricot.

Histamine: Who doesn't love apricots? Eat in moderation as higher in sugar.

Lectins: Allowed on a low-lectin diet. Best to eat when apricot is in season.

Oxalates: Low oxalate, just 5–9 mg per 100 g (Source: *University of Chicago*).

Salicylates: Apricots are thought to have a very high level of salicylates with over 1 mg per 100 g of the fruit. While they are rich in vitamin A, beta-carotene, and other carotenoids, when following a low-salicylate diet, carrots are your better bet for these nutrients. And dried apricot may be even worse. The website *Food Can Make You Ill* provides a comprehensive breakdown of an Australian study (Anne R Swain et al. Salicylates in Food. Journal of the American Dietetic Association Vol. 85:8 1985). It puts dried apricots and dates in its 'Extremely high amounts of salicylates' section.

Artichokes

- DASH: Fat: ✓ Sodium: ✓ Sugar: ✓
- Diverticulitis: Stage 1: ✗ Stage 2: ✗ Stage 3: ✓
- Histamine: ✓
- Lectin: ✓
- Oxalate: ✗
- Salicylates: 😐

DASH Diet (Hypertension): Allowed on the DASH diet. A study found artichoke leaf juice contained an antihypertensive effect in patients with mild hypertension (source: *PubMed*). *Saturated fat content: 0g (per 100g), Sodium content: 94mg (per 100g), 3% daily value based on a 2,000 calorie diet, Sugar content: 1g (per 100g).*

Diverticulitis: No solid foods can be eaten at stage one, the clear liquids diet. Allowed on the high-fiber diet.

Histamine: Acceptable.

Lectins: Contains relatively little lectin.

Oxalates: According to the University of Chicago, oxalate content of artichokes is moderate at 5 mg per one small bud.

Salicylates: Artichokes, whether they're the French or Jerusalem type, are moderately high in salicylates. According to *Healthline*, compared to other vegetables they contain some of the highest levels at .5 to 1 mg per 100 g. However, if you eat them by gently scraping off the tender bits at the bottom of the leaf, closing your teeth on it and pulling the leaf outward, rather than eating the entire heart, you may consume that small amount. (This sounds a little complicated for us!)

Artificial sweeteners

- DASH: Fat: ✓ Sodium: ✗ Sugar: ✓
- Diverticulitis: Stage 1: ✗ Stage 2: ✗ Stage 3: ✗
- Histamine: ✗
- Lectin: ✗
- Oxalate: 😕
- Salicylates: ✗

We suggest avoiding artificial sweeteners because of the potential negative effects on your gut microbiome.

DASH Diet (Hypertension): It's thought that using sugar alternatives such as stevia and splenda are acceptable on this diet but we think it is best to avoid artificial sweeteners for the reason stated above. *Saturated fat content: 0g (per 100g), Sodium content: 572mg (per 100g) 23% daily value based on a 2,000 calorie diet, Sugar content: 4g (per 100g).*

Diverticulitis: Avoid. Sweeteners may aggravate diverticulitis symptoms so they're not allowed.

Histamine: There are so many health reasons you want to be avoiding artificial sweeteners. There is much we don't know about their effects on the body. Stick to natural sweeteners like stevia.

Lectins: Very little research on lectins in artificial sweeteners; however, these should be eliminated.

Oxalates: Most sweeteners are in the category of "very low" with 0.1 - 2.9 mg of oxalates per 100 g, according to the Urology Care Foundation. We'd still urge you to avoid artificial sweeteners. Unfortunately, some natural sweeteners (which are often a better option) are higher in oxalates.

Salicylates: Plain artificial sweeteners are thought to have a low level of salicylates; however, these additives are best avoided as they can trigger symptoms similar to the adverse effects of salicylates depending on the individual. They are well-documented scientifically for the potential to cause harm to one's health, including weight gain and certain cancers.

Asparagus

- DASH: Fat: ✓ Sodium: ✓ Sugar: ✓
- Diverticulitis: Stage 1: ✗ Stage 2: 😕 Stage 3: ✓
- Histamine: ✓
- Lectin: 😕
- Oxalate: 😕
- Salicylates: 😕

DASH Diet (Hypertension): Allowed. Consume 4-5 servings of vegetables a day. *Saturated fat content: 0g (per 100g), Sodium content: 2mg (per 100g), less than 1% daily value based on a 2,000 calorie diet, Sugar content: 1.9g (per 100g).*

Diverticulitis: No solid foods can be eaten at stage one, the clear liquids diet. Only the tips are allowed on the low-fiber diet.

Histamine: Lots of veggies are great on a low-histamine diet, and asparagus is one of those.

Lectins: According to Healthline and Shawn Wells, asparagus contains relatively little lectin. Another source confirmed the lectins found in asparagus *"whether cooked or consumed raw, do not appear to cause significant GI problems"*. Test carefully.

Oxalates: Moderate in oxalates, 5 mg per 100 g (source: *University of Chicago*). According to the Oxalosis and Hyperoxaluria Foundation, asparagus contains 2 to 10 mg of oxalate in a one-half-cup serving which is also thought to be a moderate source.

Salicylates: We have looked at two types of asparagus. Canned asparagus is richer in salicylates with one 1 mg per 100 g. If you're going to eat it, choose fresh asparagus. There is some conflicting information as to the exact level of salicylates it contains, rated low to moderate depending on the source. Most reliable studies have noted that it has a low amount with levels below .25 per 100 g, but not all. Asparagus is high in folic acid and an excellent source of vitamins A, B6, C, as well as potassium and fiber.

Aubergine

- DASH: Fat: ✓ Sodium: ✓ Sugar: ✓
- Diverticulitis: Stage 1: ✗ Stage 2: 😐 Stage 3: ✓
- Histamine: ✗
- Lectin: ✗
- Oxalate: ✗
- Salicylates: ✗

Also called *eggplant*, a part of the nightshade family.

DASH Diet (Hypertension): Allowed. Consume 4-5 servings of vegetables a day. *Saturated fat content: 0g (per 100g), Sodium content: 2mg (per 100g), less than 1% daily value based on a 2,000 calorie diet, Sugar content: 3.5g (per 100g).*

Diverticulitis: No solid foods can be eaten at stage one, the clear liquids diet. Aubergines are a great source of fiber. A study found aubergines can control diabetes through their anti-oxidative properties (source: *Yarmohammadi F, Ghasemzadeh Rahbardar M, Hosseinzadeh H. Effect of eggplant (Solanum melongena) on the metabolic syndrome*). Aubergine is allowed on the high-fiber diet. Test carefully at the low-fiber stage although peeled aubergine is thought to be allowed.

Histamine: Not all veggies are created equal. Unfortunately, aubergine comes up as high in histamine on the major food lists, and many report to us their personal experience that they are not tolerated well. Fruits and vegetables with peels are often high in histamine.

Lectins: Thought to be high in lectins, particularly in the seeds and peels. So you could take the seeds and the peel off but still probably best avoided.

Oxalates: The Winchester Hospital lists eggplant in their High Oxalate, Foods To Avoid list. The PainSpy site lists Eggplant as very high. Some disagreement over oxalate content but we have listed it as high.

Salicylates: They're jam-packed with nutrients, but it also has a higher level of salicylates than many other vegetables at .5 to 1 mg per 100 g. If you consume, do so only in limited amounts. Some diets such as the Bulletproof Diet consider Aubergine to be inflammatory.

Avocado

- DASH: Fat: ✗ Sodium: ✓ Sugar: ✓
- Diverticulitis: Stage 1: ✗ Stage 2: 😐 Stage 3: ✓

- Histamine: ✗
- Lectin: ✓
- Oxalate: ✗
- Salicylates: ✗

DASH Diet (Hypertension): Allowed. Avocados are a significant source of potassium which is great for your heart. They may also lower your blood pressure (source: *Hello Heart*). Whilst avocado is healthy, it's still higher in fat compared to other fruits. *Saturated fat content: 2.1g (per 100g), Sodium content: 7mg (per 100g) less than 1% daily value based on a 2,000 calorie diet, Sugar content: 0.7g (per 100g).*

Diverticulitis: No solid foods can be eaten at stage one, the clear liquids diet. Test cautiously on the low-fiber diet.

Histamine: This is one of the major disappointments for people starting out on a low histamine diet for the first time. It almost seems incomprehensible that avocados could not be healthy. But often they are very high in histamine levels particularly ones that are very soft. Avoid or treat with extreme caution. This includes avocado oil although apparently it is lower in histamine if cold pressed.

Lectins: Full of nutrients, this superfood is thought to be low-lectin.

Oxalates: Very high in oxalates, 19 mg per 100 g (source: *The University of Chicago*).

Salicylates: Avocados tend to be on the list of foods to avoid for those with a salicylate sensitivity.

Bamboo shoots

- DASH: Fat: ✓ Sodium: ✓ Sugar: ✓
- Diverticulitis: Stage 1: ✗ Stage 2: ✗ Stage 3: ✓
- Histamine: 🤔
- Lectin: ✓
- Oxalate: ✗
- Salicylates: ✓

Note that bamboo shoots should never be eaten raw because of natural toxins present which may cause health problems (Source: *Nongdam P, Tikendra L. The Nutritional Facts of Bamboo Shoots and Their Usage as Important Traditional Foods of Northeast India*).

DASH Diet (Hypertension): Allowed. *Saturated fat content: 0.1g (per 100g), Sodium content: 4mg (per 100g) less than 1% daily value based on a 2,000 calorie diet, Sugar content: 3g (per 100g).*

Diverticulitis: No solid foods can be eaten at stage one, the clear liquids diet. Allowed on the high-fiber diet.

Histamine: Test carefully.

Lectins: Thought to be low-lectin.

Oxalates: Thought to be very high in oxalate content.

Salicylates: All reliable sources list bamboo shoots as having a low or negligible amount of salicylates. Highly nutritious, they're a wonderful source of vitamins B6 and E, fiber, and copper.

Banana

- DASH: Fat: ✓ Sodium: ✓ Sugar: ✗
- Diverticulitis: Stage 1: ✗ Stage 2: 🤔 Stage 3: ✓
- Histamine: ✗

- Lectin: 🤢
- Oxalate: ✓
- Salicylates: ✓

DASH Diet (Hypertension): Low in saturated fat and sodium content but high in sugar. Eat in moderation. *Saturated fat content: 0.1g (per 100g), Sodium content: 1mg (per 100g), Sugar content: 12g (per 100g).*

Diverticulitis: No solid foods can be eaten at stage one, the clear liquids diet. Only ripe bananas are allowed on the low-fiber diet.

Histamine: Bananas can often be very high in histamine. It's thought that the younger/greener, the better you will tolerate it, so avoid ripe bananas.

Lectins: Bananas vary massively by ripeness. Avoid ripe bananas. Instead, go for green bananas which are safe to eat on a low-lectin diet. Studies have also shown that lectins from bananas become more potent after heating (source: *https://dadamo.com/txt/index.pl?1007*) therefore, cooking or baking bananas should also be avoided.

Oxalates: Low oxalate, just 5–9 mg per 100 g (source: *University of Chicago*).

Salicylates: Lots of fruits are frustratingly high in salicylates, but not bananas. Bananas are very low in salicylates with less than .1 mg per 100 g. They contain a significant amount of vitamin B6 and potassium and other nutrients.

Barley

- DASH: Fat: ✓ Sodium: ✓ Sugar: ✓
- Diverticulitis: Stage 1: ✗ Stage 2: ✗ Stage 3: ✓
- Histamine: 🤢
- Lectin: ✗
- Oxalate: ✓
- Salicylates: ✓

DASH Diet (Hypertension): Allowed. Evidence shows Barley reduces blood pressure (source: *Oldways Whole Grains Council*). *Saturated fat content: 0.5g (per 100g), Sodium content: 12mg (per 100g), less than 1% daily value based on a 2,000 calorie diet, Sugar content: 0.8g (per 100g).*

Diverticulitis: No solid foods can be eaten at stage one, the clear liquids diet. Allowed on the high-fiber diet.

Histamine: Barley seems to be tolerated well. However, it contains gluten and many people who are low histamine will follow a gluten-free diet and therefore will want to avoid barley.

Lectins: High in lectins. One to put in your 'avoid' list.

Oxalates: 3.0 - 4.9 mg per 100 g, low oxalate (source: *Open Nutrition Journal*).

Salicylates: Barley isn't gluten-free, but it is considered a healthy whole grain that contains only a negligible amount of salicylates. To avoid additives (which might change the salicylate content), use it as an ingredient in homemade bread.

Barley malt, malt

- DASH: Fat: ✓ Sodium: ✓ Sugar: ✓
- Diverticulitis: Stage 1: ✗ Stage 2: ✗ Stage 3: ✓
- Histamine: ✗
- Lectin: ✗

- Oxalate: ✗
- Salicylates: ✗

A natural sweetener from barley.

DASH Diet (Hypertension): This is a great substitute for sugar and allowed on the DASH diet. *Saturated fat content: 0.4g (per 100g), Sodium content: 11mg (per 100g) less than 1% daily value based on a 2,000 calorie diet, Sugar content: 0.8g (per 100g).*

Diverticulitis: Allowed on the high-fiber diet.

Histamine: Different from barley as fermented, which is a big no-no in histamine.

Lectins: Considered a whole grain. Avoid as high in lectins.

Oxalates: High, best avoided.

Salicylates: A rich source of soluble fiber, malt extract is also low in salicylates.

Basil

- DASH: Fat: ✓ Sodium: ✓ Sugar: ✓
- Diverticulitis: Stage 1: 😐 Stage 2: ✓ Stage 3: ✓
- Histamine: ✓
- Lectin: ✓
- Oxalate: ✓
- Salicylates: ✓

DASH Diet (Hypertension): Allowed. PubMed has published a study on the role of herbs in treating hypertension. They found basil causes a fall in systolic, diastolic, and mean blood pressure *(source: Tabassum N, Ahmad F. Role of natural herbs in the treatment of hypertension. Pharmacogn Rev). Saturated fat content: 0g (per 100g), Sodium content: 4mg (per 100g) less than 1% daily value based on a 2,000 calorie diet, Sugar content: 0.3g (per 100g).*

Diverticulitis: Allowed on the low-fiber diet. Go for basil seeds if you want higher fiber content.

Histamine: Delicious. We love making basil pesto with olive oil and a small amount of almonds.

Lectins: Thought to be low-lectin.

Oxalates: Not a massive amount of information out there, but UPMC lists them as low-oxalate. We love making basil pesto with olive oil and a few almonds.

Salicylates: Our research suggests basil is a herb that contains one of the highest levels of salicylates. While the number of milligrams is not available because of limited research, avoid or proceed with caution, using only a small amount.

Beans

- DASH: Fat: ✓ Sodium: ✓ Sugar: ✓
- Diverticulitis: Stage 1: ✗ Stage 2: ✗ Stage 3: ✓
- Histamine: ✗
- Lectin: ✗
- Oxalate: ✗
- Salicylates: 😐

DASH Diet (Hypertension): Allowed. Ensure you eat only 4-5 servings a week. *Saturated fat content: 0.2g (per 100g), Sodium content: 12mg (per 100g), less than 1% daily value based on a 2,000 calorie diet, Sugar content: 2.1g (per 100g).*

Diverticulitis: No solid foods can be eaten at stage one, the clear liquids diet. Allowed on the high-fiber diet.

Histamine: Ugh, beans and histamine intolerance rarely go together. Everybody is different and there may be exceptions but we rarely react well to them.

Lectins: High in lectins (including borlotti beans, broad beans and green beans). One to put in your 'avoid' list. If you want to eat beans, the FDA recommends boiling them for 30 minutes to reduce lectin content. Avoid canned beans as most of these have not been soaked or cooked to reduce lectin content. As previously reiterated, soaking may reduce lectin content.

Oxalates: Beans are high in oxalates. Kidney beans could be a better option with about 15 mg per half a cup, but beans generally = oxalates (source: *North Dakota State University*).

Salicylates: Beans and salicylates are a little complicated. When is it ever not complicated with salicylates? Most beans contain only trace amounts; however French beans may have up to .25 mg per 100 g. Avoid or limit broad and fava beans which have a higher level.

Beef

- DASH: Fat: ✗ Sodium: ✓ Sugar: ✓
- Diverticulitis: Stage 1: ✗ Stage 2: ✓ Stage 3: ✓
- Histamine: ✓
- Lectin: ✓
- Oxalate: ✓
- Salicylates: ✓

DASH Diet (Hypertension): Must be grass-fed beef as grain-fed beef contributes to inflammation and heart disease (source: *Medicine Net*). Eat no more than 2 servings a day. *Saturated fat content: 6g (per 100g), Sodium content: 72mg (per 100g), 3% daily value based on a 2,000 calorie diet, Sugar content: 0g (per 100g).*

Diverticulitis: No solid foods can be eaten at stage one, the clear liquids diet. Allowed on the low-fiber diet.

Histamine: There are a few rules here. It should be organic - in fact it must be, so that you avoid fertilizers and pesticides. It's also – and this is the big issue – must not be aged. Next time you are in a steak restaurant to take a close look at the menu. You'll see that most of the cuts of meat on there are actually aged and therefore will be high and histamine. However, if you can find some fresh beef that is organic then you are good to go.

Lectins: Beef may be eaten on a low-lectin diet. Avoid corn-fed beef and opt for grass-fed for general health reasons.

Oxalates: Meats are normally safe to eat on a low-oxalate diet. Remember, eating large portions of meat is thought to potentially increase the risk of kidney stones.

Salicylates: See "Meat"

Beer

- DASH: Fat: ✓ Sodium: ✓ Sugar: ✓
- Diverticulitis: Stage 1: ✗ Stage 2: ✗ Stage 3: ✗
- Histamine: ✗
- Lectin: ✗

- Oxalate: ✓
- Salicylates: ✗

DASH Diet (Hypertension): Drink alcohol sparingly on the DASH diet. You don't have to eliminate alcohol completely although it's good to limit consumption. *Saturated fat content: 0g (per 100g), Sodium content: 4mg less than 1% daily value based on a 2,000 calorie diet, Sugar content: 0g (per 100g).*

Diverticulitis: See "Alcohol."

Histamine: See "Alcohol."

Lectins: Avoid them as it's thought to be high in lectins.

Oxalates: See "Alcohol."

Salicylates: Beer contains a high level of salicylates.

Beetroot

- DASH: Fat: ✓ Sodium: ✓ Sugar: ✗
- Diverticulitis: Stage 1: ✗ Stage 2: ✓ Stage 3: ✓
- Histamine: ✓
- Lectin: ✓
- Oxalate: ✗
- Salicylates: 🤔
- Also known as *Beets*.

DASH Diet (Hypertension): This lovely veg contains nitrates — natural chemicals which help promote blood flow. Studies have shown nitrates *"acutely lowers blood pressure"*. Consume 4-5 servings of vegetables a day. *Saturated fat content: 0g (per 100g), Sodium content: 78mg (per 100g), 3% daily value based on a 2,000 calorie diet, Sugar content: 7g (per 100g).*

Diverticulitis: No solid foods can be eaten at stage one, the clear liquids diet. Allowed on the low-fiber diet if cooked.

Histamine: Acceptable.

Lectins: Kimberly Gomer, Director of Nutrition at the Pritikin Longevity Center in Miami confirmed the lectins found in beets *"whether cooked or consumed raw, do not appear to cause significant GI problems"*. The best way to keep the nutrients is to gently sautéed, steam or roast them (source: *Stacy Mitchell Doyle, M.D., founder of FoodTherapyMD.com*).

Oxalates: Very high in oxalates - one of the highest foods around. The website Healthline notes; *"Levels of oxalates are much higher in the leaves than the root itself, but the root is considered high in oxalates"*.

Salicylates: It is difficult to definitely rate beetroot. We have come across a lot of conflicting research. Based on this divergence of opinion, test carefully and we believe it may be best to avoid canned beetroot and choose fresh, proceeding with caution. Let's explain in a little more detail. There is some debate as to the level of salicylates in beetroot. According to research published in the Journal of the American Dietetic Association, fresh beets have just .18 mg per 100 g. Canned beets are higher, with a moderate amount of up to .49 mg per 100 g. When we dig into our sources, Millhouse Medical Centre categorizes beets as moderate, while Drugs.com puts beetroot in the "high" category, and the other lists also cannot quite agree. So... as always, proceed carefully and find your individual tolerance level.

Bell pepper (hot or sweet)

- DASH: Fat: ✓ Sodium: ✓ Sugar: ✓
- Diverticulitis: Stage 1: ✗ Stage 2: 😐 Stage 3: ✓
- Histamine: 😐
- Lectin: ✗
- Oxalate: Sweet: 😐 Hot: ✗
- Salicylates: ✗

A great source of vitamin C. Half a cup of raw red pepper is thought to contain 95 mg of vitamin C, which is 106% of the daily value (source: *Medical News Today*)

DASH Diet (Hypertension): Allowed. *Saturated fat content: 0g (per 100g), Sodium content: 9mg (per 100g), less than 1% daily value based on a 2,000 calorie diet, Sugar content: 5g (per 100g).*

Diverticulitis: No solid foods can be eaten at stage one, the clear liquids diet. Test cautiously on the low-fiber diet and must be cooked.

Histamine: Some may be okay with hot bell peppers. Test very carefully. Sweet bell pepper is high in pesticide residue according to Mast Cell 360, buy organic. (This applies really to all foods - but especially foods which collect more pesticide. We tend to buy all our produce organic, which means we'll never be rich, but we will be healthier!)

Lectins: Part of the nightshade family which are high in lectins particularly in the seeds and peels.

Oxalates: Hot chili pepper is often categorized as high, 10.0-14.9 mg (source: *Harvard*). Sweet pepper is thought to be moderate in oxalates, but it can be very high in pesticide residue.

Salicylates: Hot peppers are very high in salicylates although the capsaicin they contain may reduce adverse effects. Consume minimally until you know how your body will react. Sweet bell peppers also have a high level of salicylates. Avoid sweet peppers which contain a high level of salicylates without the capsaicin.

Bison

- DASH: Fat: ✓ Sodium: ✓ Sugar: ✓
- Diverticulitis: Stage 1: ✗ Stage 2: ✓ Stage 3: ✗
- Histamine: ✓
- Lectin: ✓
- Oxalate: ✓
- Salicylates: ✓

DASH Diet (Hypertension): Allowed. The American Heart Association also recommends bison. Consume no more than 2 servings a day. *Saturated fat content: 0.69g (per 100g), Sodium content: 54mg (per 100g) 2% daily value based on a 2,000 calorie diet, Sugar content: 0g (per 100g)* (source: *Fatsecret Platform API*).

Diverticulitis: No solid foods can be eaten at stage one, the clear liquids diet. Bison contains no fiber so they're allowed on the low-fiber diet.

Histamine: Must not be aged. Same as beef, high in histamine if aged. We would love to eat more bison but struggle to source it where we live. It's an excellent alternative to beef with less saturated fat.

Lectins: Thought to be low-lectin. Opt for grass-fed bison.

Oxalates: Most meats are low in oxalates. We would love to eat more bison but struggle to source it where we live. It's a good alternative to beef with less saturated fat although we have struggled to find much specific information on oxalates. It is likely low oxalate but as always, test carefully. Remember, eating large portions of meat is thought to potentially increase the risk of kidney stones.

Salicylates: Meat is salicylate-free, and bison can be a suitable alternative to beef as it contains less saturated fat and is lower in calories.

While it's more expensive, grass-fed bison is best. Traditionally farmed options cost less but have a different nutritional profile as multiple studies have noted.

Bivalves (mussels, oysters, clams, scallops)

- DASH:
  - Mussels: Fat: ✓ Sodium: ✗ Sugar: ✓
  - Oysters: Fat: ✗ Sodium: ✗ Sugar: ✓
  - Clams: Fat: ✓ Sodium: ✗ Sugar: ✓
  - Scallops: Fat: ✓ Sodium: ✗ Sugar: ✓
- Diverticulitis: Stage 1: ✗ Stage 2: ✓ Stage 3: ✗
- Histamine: ✗
- Lectin: 😐
- Oxalate: ✓
- Salicylates: ✓

Who knew these kinds of seafood were called bivalves?

DASH Diet (Hypertension): Mussels, clams and scallops are high in sodium. Oysters are low in sugar but thought to be high in saturated fat and sodium content. Avoid. **Mussels**: *Saturated fat content: 0.9g (per 100g), Sodium content: 369 mg (per 100g) 15% daily value based on a 2,000 calorie diet, Sugar content: 0g (per 100g).* **Oysters**: *Saturated fat content: 3.2g (per 100g), Sodium content: 417mg (per 100g) 17% daily value based on a 2,000 calorie diet, Sugar content: 0g (per 100g).* **Clams** (source: nutritionix): *Saturated fat content: 0.2g (per 100g), Sodium content: 1,202mg (per 100g), 50% daily value based on a 2,000 calorie diet, Sugar content: 0g (per 100g).* **Scallops**: *Saturated fat content: 0.2g (per 100g), Sodium content: 667mg (per 100g), 27% daily value based on a 2,000 calorie diet, Sugar content: 0g (per 100g).*

Diverticulitis: No solid foods can be eaten at stage one, the clear liquids diet. Allowed on the low-fiber diet.

Histamine: Bad news for seafood lovers.

Lectins: A study found lectins present in bivalves (source: *ResearchGate: Lectins with Varying Specificity and Biological Activity from Marine Bivalves*) however, we're not sure of the lectin levels. Having studied the limited available research we'd ask you to test carefully.

Oxalates: Thought to be low oxalate.

Salicylates: Thankfully, they are a low salicylate food.

Black caraway

- DASH: Fat: ✓ Sodium: ✓ Sugar: ✓
- Diverticulitis: Stage 1: ✗ Stage 2: ✗ Stage 3: ✓
- Histamine: ✓
- Lectin: 😐
- Oxalate: ✗
- Salicylates: ✗

DASH Diet (Hypertension): Allowed. *Saturated fat content: 0.5g (per 100g), Sodium content: 88 mg (per 100g), 3% daily value based on a 2,000 calorie diet, Sugar content: 0.64g (per 100g).*

Diverticulitis: No solid foods can be eaten at stage one, the clear liquids diet. Allowed on the high-fiber diet.

Histamine: One of the good guys... can help lower histamine levels.

Lectins: It's unclear whether black caraway seeds are high in lectins but we know that caraway seeds are a source of lectins (source: *Functional Nutrition Library*). Test carefully.

Oxalates: According to research, extensive amounts of total oxalate (201-4014 mg/100 g D.W.) were found in daily common herbs such as caraway seed, green cardamom, cinnamon, coriander seeds, cumin, curry powder, ginger, and turmeric powder (source: *The Canadian Center of Science and Education*). Depends on the quantities used.

Salicylates: Black caraway is categorized as high in salicylates, and we'll put it in a category below "very high." After some extensive digging we could not find definitive information on the exact salicylate content, however we feel this spice should be limited or avoided altogether.

Blackberry

- DASH: Fat: ✓ Sodium: ✓ Sugar: ✓
- Diverticulitis: Stage 1: ✗ Stage 2: ✗ Stage 3: ✓
- Histamine: ✓
- Lectin: 🤔
- Oxalate: 🤔
- Salicylates: ✗

DASH Diet (Hypertension): Allowed. This superfood is great for the brain and helps reduce blood pressure (source: *Urology of Virginia*). *Saturated fat content: 0g (per 100g), Sodium content: 1mg (per 100g) less than 1% daily value based on a 2,000 calorie diet, Sugar content: 4.9g (per 100g).*

Diverticulitis: No solid foods can be eaten at stage one, the clear liquids diet. Allowed on the high-fiber diet.

Histamine: Allowed.

Lectins: Mixed opinions on this one, as with so much in the lectin world.

One source confirms blackberries are a source of lectins. In Nathan Sharon's book Lectins, he confirmed that blackberries *"exhibit lectin activity"*. However, other sources disagree. Best to eat when blackberries are in season (source: *Health Canal*). Test carefully.

Oxalates: Blueberries and blackberries have just 4 mg per cup (source: *North Dakota State University*). Also rich in antioxidants.

Salicylates: Blackberries are rich in antioxidants, but they contain an outrageous amount of salicylates with over 1 mg per 100 g.

Blackcurrants

- DASH: Fat: ✓ Sodium: ✓ Sugar: ✓
- Diverticulitis: Stage 1: ✗ Stage 2: ✗ Stage 3: ✓
- Histamine: ✓
- Lectin: ✗
- Oxalate: ✗
- Salicylates: ✗

Also known as *currants*.

DASH Diet (Hypertension): Allowed. Try not to eat too much if you're also taking medication to lower blood pressure because blackcurrants may lower your blood pressure further (source: *webMD*). *Saturated fat content: 0.034g (per 100g), Sodium content: 2mg (per 100g) less than 1% daily value based on a 2,000 calorie diet, Sugar content: 0g (per 100g).*

Diverticulitis: No solid foods can be eaten at stage one, the clear liquids diet. A superb source of fiber, allowed on the high-fiber diet.

Histamine: Acceptable.

Lectins: Thought to be a source of lectins.

Oxalates: Moderate in oxalates, should be limited.

Salicylates: Blackcurrants are usually cooked in savory or sweet dishes, and used to make syrup, preserves, or jam. Unfortunately, they have a high level of salicylates, so mostly avoid or consume them minimally with caution, and be aware of their presence in other dishes.

Blue cheeses

- DASH: Fat: ✗ Sodium: ✗ Sugar: ✓
- Diverticulitis: Stage 1: ✗ Stage 2: ✓ Stage 3: ✗
- Histamine: ✗
- Lectin: 😕
- Oxalate: ✓
- Salicylates: 😕

DASH Diet (Hypertension): Low in sugar but thought to be high in saturated fat and sodium content. Avoid. *Saturated fat content: 19g (per 100g), Sodium content: 1,395mg (per 100g), 58% daily value based on a 2,000 calorie diet, Sugar content: 0.5g (per 100g).*

Diverticulitis: No solid foods can be eaten at stage one, the clear liquids diet. Blue cheese contains no fiber so they're allowed on the low-fiber diet.

Histamine: These blue cheeses are blue because they are moldy and therefore high in histamine. There are other cheese options which are lower histamine and you can find them throughout this book. Take a look at ricotta cheese, cream cheese and soft cheese. You might also get on well with mozzarella.

Lectins: Cheese acquires lectins from the molds that grow within it (source: *Understanding Arthritis, The Clinical Way Forward by W. Fox, D. Freed*). Test carefully as molds are used in blue cheese production.

Oxalates: Dairy is free of oxalate. It's also high in calcium, so it is a good choice, although cheese can have other health implications. What about dressings? Blue cheese dressing has less than 5 mg of oxalates per 100 g (source: *Urinary Stones - The Oxalate Content Of Food*).

Salicylates: While most cheeses have negligible amounts of salicylates, blue cheese contains a moderate amount and should be limited in consumption despite containing more calcium than other types.

Blue fenugreek

- DASH: No information
- Diverticulitis: Stage 1: ✗ Stage 2: ✗ Stage 3: 😕
- Histamine: ✓
- Lectin: 😕
- Oxalate: ✗

- Salicylates: ✗

Diverticulitis: Fenugreek is high in fiber so we think blue fenugreek could be high in fiber too. Avoid blue fenugreek at the clear liquid and the low-fiber stages of the diet.

Histamine: Acceptable.

Lectins: Blue fenugreek has a milder, less bitter taste than normal fenugreek. There is a limited amount of lectin research on blue fenugreek, but there are lectins present in fenugreek (source: *Food and Nutrition Journal*).

Oxalates: Very high; total oxalate of blue fenugreek powder amounted to 1246 mg/100 g. (source: *Scientific Electronic Library Online of Brazil*).

Salicylates: Blue fenugreek, widely used in Georgian cuisine, is very high in salicylates with at least 1 mg per 100 g.

Blueberries

- DASH: Fat: ✓ Sodium: ✓ Sugar: ✓
- Diverticulitis: Stage 1: ✗ Stage 2: ✗ Stage 3: ✓
- Histamine: ✓
- Lectin: 😐
- Oxalate: 😐
- Salicylates: ✗

DASH Diet (Hypertension): Allowed. Harvard's website notes: "*Consuming 200 grams of blueberries (about one cup) daily can improve blood vessel function and decrease systolic blood pressure.*" Saturated fat content: 0g (per 100g), Sodium content: 1mg (per 100g) less than 1% daily value based on a 2,000 calorie diet, Sugar content: 10g (per 100g).

Diverticulitis: No solid foods can be eaten at stage one, the clear liquids diet. Allowed on the high-fiber diet.

Histamine: Some say blueberries are histamine fighting, which is good news.

Lectin: Mixed opinion. Some sources confirm blueberries do not contain lectins whereas other sources say blueberries contain relatively little lectin. Test carefully. As with all fruits, it's best to eat when blueberries are in season. A study found "*a lack of the antinutrient lectins*" in Andean blueberries (source: *Baenas N, Ruales J, Moreno DA, Barrio DA, Stinco CM, Martínez-Cifuentes G, Meléndez-Martínez AJ, García-Ruiz A. Characterization of Andean Blueberry in Bioactive Compounds, Evaluation of Biological Properties, and In Vitro Bioaccessibility*).

Oxalates: Blueberries and blackberries have 4 mg per cup (source: *a publication by North Dakota State University*). Blueberries are also rich in antioxidants, which can help ward off cancer, heart disease, and other serious health conditions.

Salicylates: Blueberries are very high in salicylates, but they are also an extremely rich source of antioxidants which can lower the risk of serious health conditions like heart disease and cancer. Rather than avoid them altogether, consume on a limited basis.

Bok choi

- DASH: Fat: ✓ Sodium: ✓ Sugar: ✓
- Diverticulitis: Stage 1: ✗ Stage 2: ✗ Stage 3: ✓
- Histamine: ✓
- Lectin: ✓
- Oxalate: ✓
- Salicylates: 😐

Sometimes also written as *bok choy*. A type of Chinese white cabbage in the cruciferous family, it's very high in vitamin C. Try sautéing or lightly roasting for 15 minutes if welcomed on the diet.

DASH Diet (Hypertension): Researchers found sulforaphane (the active ingredient in bok choi) helps to reduce blood pressure (source: *OHSU Research News*). Allowed. *Saturated fat content: 0g (per 100g), Sodium content: 65mg (per 100g), 2% daily value based on a 2,000 calorie diet, Sugar content: 1.2g.*

Diverticulitis: No solid foods can be eaten at stage one, the clear liquids diet. Allowed on the high-fiber diet.

Histamine: Acceptable.

Lectins: Falls under the cruciferous vegetable family (includes broccoli, kale, cabbage, radish etc.). These are thought to be low-lectin and rich in vitamin C, folate and fiber.

Oxalates: Thought to be very low in oxalates - only around 1 mg per 100 g.

Salicylates: Also spelled as bok choy, our research has found that this leafy green vegetable has a moderate amount of salicylates, from .25 to .49 mg per 100 g.

Borlotti beans

- DASH: Fat: ✓ Sodium: ✓ Sugar: ✓
- Diverticulitis: Stage 1: ✗ Stage 2: ✗ Stage 3: ✓
- Histamine: ✗
- Lectin: ✗
- Oxalate: ✗
- Salicylates: 😐

Also known as the *cranberry bean*.

DASH Diet (Hypertension): Allowed but ensure you eat only 4-5 servings a week. *Saturated fat content: 0.3g (per 100g), Sodium content: 0mg (per 100g), Sugar content: 0.83g (per 100g).*

Diverticulitis: No solid foods can be eaten at stage one, the clear liquids diet. Allowed on the high-fiber diet.

Histamine: See our more general comments under *Beans*.

Lectins: High in lectins. One to put in your 'avoid' list. If you want to consume beans, the FDA recommends boiling them for 30 minutes to reduce lectin content. Avoid canned beans as most of these have not been soaked or cooked to reduce lectin content.

Oxalates: See our more general comments under *Beans*.

Salicylates: See "Beans" for more information.

Bouillon

- DASH: Fat: ✗ Sodium: ✗ Sugar: ✗
- Diverticulitis: Stage 1: ✓ Stage 2: ✓ Stage 3: ✗
- Histamine: ✗
- Lectin: 😐
- Oxalate: 😐
- Salicylates: ✗

Also known as *broth*.

DASH Diet (Hypertension): Broth is made from simmering water with either meat, fish or seafood. It's very high in sodium so avoid it. *Saturated fat content: 3.4g (per 100g), Sodium content: 23,875mg (per 100g) 994% daily value based on a 2,000 calorie diet, Sugar content: 17g (per 100g)*

Diverticulitis: Bouillon contains no fiber, so they're allowed on the clear liquid diet and low-fiber diet.

Histamine: Stocks are often high histamine if they're bone broth. In addition, shop-bought ones can be a lot worse. According to SIGHI, its ingredients are almost always incompatible (glutamate, yeast extract, spice/ aroma/ flavor/ seasoning/ condiment, meat extracts, incompatible vegetables)

Lectins: Broth is made from simmering water with either meat, fish or seafood. The amount of lectins depends on the type of broth. Shop-bought stocks and bouillons can have a lot of different ingredients, so it's always worth checking closely. Very difficult to give a rating as there's very little research after careful analysis. Test carefully.

Oxalates: Very difficult to give a rating for the reasons stated above.

Salicylates: Very difficult to give a rating for the reasons stated above but the most reliable lists rank them as high in salicylates. Another negative, they contain flavor enhancers and other unhealthy ingredients like monosodium glutamate.

Boysenberry

- DASH: Fat: ✔ Sodium: ✔ Sugar: ✔
- Diverticulitis: Stage 1: ✘ Stage 2: ✘ Stage 3: ✔
- Histamine: 😐
- Lectin: 😐
- Oxalate: ✔
- Salicylates: ✘

A cross of loganberry, blackberry and raspberry. Boysenberries offer a slew of minerals like potassium, iron, calcium, and manganese.

DASH Diet (Hypertension): As potassium and magnesium has been found to reduce blood pressure it is allowed. *Saturated fat content: 0.014g (per 100g), Sodium content: 0mg (per 100g), Sugar content: 4.88g (per 100g)* (source: *Fatsecret Platform API*).

Diverticulitis: No solid foods can be eaten at stage one, the clear liquids diet. Allowed on the high-fiber diet.

Histamine: Test carefully.

Lectins: Given that loganberry, blackberry and raspberry all contain lectins, we think there are moderate amounts of lectin in boysenberries. Test carefully.

Oxalates: Low; 2-6 mg/100g (source: *Journal of Food Composition and Analysis*).

Salicylates: They contain a very high level of salicylates, with at least 1 mg per 100 g. Avoid or consume with caution in limited amounts.

Brandy

- DASH: Fat: ✔ Sodium: ✔ Sugar: ✔
- Diverticulitis: Stage 1: ✘ Stage 2: ✘ Stage 3: ✘
- Histamine: ✘
- Lectin: 😐
- Oxalate: ✔

- Salicylates: ✗

A distilled liquor made from fermented fruit juice or wine (source: *Whiskey Bon*).

DASH Diet (Hypertension): Whilst brandy is allowed on the DASH diet, as with all alcohol, drink in moderation as too much alcohol will raise blood pressure. *Saturated fat content: 0g (per 100g), Sodium content: 1mg (per 100g), less than 1% daily value based on a 2,000 calorie diet, Sugar content: 0g (per 100g).*

Diverticulitis: See "Alcohol"

Histamine: See "Alcohol"

Lectins: It's not clear-cut whether brandy should be avoided as brandy can be made from a range of fruits from grapes to pears, raspberries, apples, cherries, etc. The lectin content could depend on the type of fruit used during the process. As with all alcohol, consume in moderation and test carefully. Very difficult to give a rating.

Oxalates: See "Alcohol"

Salicylates: Alcoholic beverages like beer, wine, and spirits such as rum and sherry contain a high level of salicylates. Champagne and sparkling wine are on the higher end, with Drambuie containing one of the highest levels for a liqueur. Dry, white wines have a lower amount while beer and ale can range anywhere from .32 to 1.26 per 100 g. Of course, there are also the other negative health effects of alcohol to consider.

Brazil nut

- DASH: Fat: ✗ Sodium: ✓ Sugar: ✓
- Diverticulitis: Stage 1: ✗ Stage 2: ✗ Stage 3: ✓
- Histamine: ✓
- Lectin: ✓
- Oxalate: ✗
- Salicylates: 😐

DASH Diet (Hypertension): They're also high in potassium. Ensure you eat only 4-5 servings a week and go for unsalted nuts. *Saturated fat content: 15g (per 100g), Sodium content: 3mg (per 100g) less than 1% daily value based on a 2,000 calorie diet, Sugar content: 2.3g (per 100g).*

Diverticulitis: No solid foods can be eaten at stage one, the clear liquids diet. Allowed on the high-fiber diet.

Histamine: Certain nuts can be high in histamine if moldy, but brazil nuts should be okay.

Lectins: Acceptable on a low-lectin diet.

Oxalates: Pine nuts, candlenuts, and Brazil nuts contain high levels of gastric soluble oxalate (492.0–556.8 mg/100 g). The intestinal soluble oxalate is the fraction that will be absorbed in the small intestine. (source: *Journal of Food Composition and Analysis*)

Salicylates: Brazil nuts contain a moderate amount of salicylates, ranging from .25 to .49 mg per 100 g. They are quite high in selenium which offers potent antioxidant properties to reduce inflammation and support heart health; however, it's important not to consume too many (which is difficult) as this quickly raises the salicylate content.

Bread

- DASH: Fat: ✓ Sodium: ✗ Sugar: ✓
- Diverticulitis: Stage 1: ✗ Stage 2: 😐 Stage 3: ✓
- Histamine: 😐

- Lectin: ✗
- Oxalate: 😖
- Salicylates: 😖

DASH Diet (Hypertension): High in sodium. Unfortunately, this staple food is the top contributor of dietary sodium in the US (source: *Vox*). Limit intake. *Saturated fat content: 0.7g (per 100g), Sodium content: 491mg, 20% daily value based on a 2,000 calorie diet (per 100g), Sugar content: 5g (per 100g).*

Diverticulitis: No solid foods can be eaten at stage one, the clear liquids diet. Go for white bread only on the low-fiber diet. Brown bread is rich in fiber.

Histamine: As we don't know the ingredients of each individual bread, check the individual ingredients on our list in this book. Also, the fermentation process and yeasting process is uncertain but you may well tolerate most breads. Test with caution. You could even make your own!

Lectins: High in lectins. One to put in your 'avoid' list.

Oxalates: Check the individual ingredients on our list in this book. On close inspection of oxalate lists, corn and oatmeal bread are thought to be lower oxalate than wheat bread. Also, the fermentation process and yeasting process is uncertain but you may well tolerate most breads. Test with caution. That said, drugs.com notes these breads are low-to-medium oxalate foods to include in the diet: *"White bread, cornbread, bagels, and white English muffins (medium oxalate). In sum, breads can range from very high in oxalates (French toast with 13 mg per two slices) to low (oat bran, corn, and oatmeal bread with 4 mg per slice/piece)."*

Salicylates: Check ingredients individually for reasons stated above. The manufacturing process typically includes emulsifiers and cutting oils along with other processing aids that can contain salicylates. Many people with a salicylate sensitivity can tolerate most breads, but to be sure you might want to make your own using low-salicylate ingredients. Time-consuming, we know…

Broad-leaved garlic

- DASH: Fat: ✓ Sodium: ✓ Sugar: ✓
- Diverticulitis: Stage 1: ✗ Stage 2: 😖 Stage 3: ✓
- Histamine: 😖
- Lectin: ✓
- Oxalate: ✓
- Salicylates: No information

Also known as *wild garlic*.

DASH Diet (Hypertension): We've used the nutritional values for garlic as the USDA and other sources do not list the nutritional values for broad-leaved garlic. Allowed and consume 4-5 servings of vegetables a day. *Saturated fat content: 0.089g (per 100g), Sodium content: 17mg (per 100g), 1% daily value based on a 2,000 calorie diet, Sugar content: 1g (per 100g).*

Diverticulitis: No solid foods can be eaten at stage one, the clear liquids diet. Test cautiously on the low-fiber diet.

Histamine: Test carefully.

Lectins: Given that garlic is acceptable on a low-lectin diet, broad-leaved garlic may be too.

Oxalates: All kinds of garlic, raw or cooked, are very low in oxalates (less than 5mg per 100 g).

Broad beans

- DASH: Fat: ✓ Sodium: ✓ Sugar: ✗
- Diverticulitis: Stage 1: ✗ Stage 2: ✗ Stage 3: ✓
- Histamine: ✗
- Lectin: ✗
- Oxalate: ✗
- Salicylates: ✗

Also known as *Vicia Faba*.

DASH Diet (Hypertension): Low in saturated fat and sodium content but high in sugar. Eat in moderation. Ensure you eat only 4-5 servings a week. *Saturated fat content: 0.1g (per 100g), Sodium content: 25mg (per 100g), 1% daily value based on a 2,000 calorie diet, Sugar content: 9g (per 100g).*

Diverticulitis: No solid foods can be eaten at stage one, the clear liquids diet. Allowed on the high-fiber diet.

Histamine: See comments on "Beans".

Lectins: These are high in lectins. One to put in your 'avoid' list. If you want to eat beans, the FDA recommends boiling them for 30 minutes to reduce lectin content. Avoid canned beans as most of these have not been soaked or cooked to reduce lectin content (source: *The Woodlands Institute*).

Oxalates: See "Beans" for details.

Salicylates: Avoid or limit broad beans which are high.

Broccoli

- DASH: Fat: ✓ Sodium: ✓ Sugar: ✓
- Diverticulitis: Stage 1: ✗ Stage 2: ✗ Stage 3: ✓
- Histamine: ✓
- Lectin: ✓
- Oxalate: 😖
- Salicylates: ✗

Rich in vitamin C, folate and fiber and falls under the cruciferous vegetable family (includes Brussels sprouts, kale, cabbage, radish etc.).

DASH Diet (Hypertension): Allowed. Researchers found sulforaphane (the active ingredient in broccoli) helps to reduce blood pressure (source: *OHSU Research News*). Consume 4-5 servings of vegetables a day. *Saturated fat content: 0.039g (per 100g), Sodium content: 33mg (per 100g) less than 1% daily value based on a 2,000 calorie diet, Sugar content: 1.7g (per 100g)* (source: *Fatsecret Platform API*).

Diverticulitis: No solid foods can be eaten at stage one, the clear liquids diet. Allowed on the high-fiber diet.

Histamine: So good for you. Enjoy.

Lectins: These are thought to be low-lectin.

Oxalates: According to the University of Chicago, half a cup of chopped broccoli has 6 mg of oxalates, which is moderate. The Pain Spy website considers broccoli to have 190 mg of oxalates per 100g.

Salicylates: Broccoli offers a lot in nutrition, including more protein than most vegetables, along with fiber, vitamins C and K, but it contains reasonably high levels of salicylates depending on the source, however, you might find that you do okay with a small amount.

Brussels sprouts

- DASH: Fat: ✓ Sodium: ✓ Sugar: ✓
- Diverticulitis: Stage 1: ✗ Stage 2: ✗ Stage 3: ✓
- Histamine: 🤔
- Lectin: ✓
- Oxalate: ✗
- Salicylates: ✓

DASH Diet (Hypertension): Allowed. One cup of Brussels sprouts contains roughly 350mg of potassium (source: *Unity Point*). Eat 4-5 servings of vegetables a day. *Saturated fat content: 0.1g (per 100g), Sodium content: 25mg (per 100g), 1% daily value based on a 2,000 calorie diet, Sugar content: 2.2g (per 100g).*

Diverticulitis: No solid foods can be eaten at stage one, the clear liquids diet. Allowed on the high-fiber diet.

Histamine: Some say Brussels sprouts are low histamine so it's very much worth testing them out. We like to buy them and freeze them and cook from frozen in the oven.

Lectins: Falls under the cruciferous vegetable family (includes broccoli, kale, cabbage, radish etc.). Again, these are thought to be low-lectin and rich in vitamin C, folate and fiber.

Oxalates: Thought to be high in oxalates. Avoid.

Salicylates: Brussels sprouts are low in salicylates and rich in vitamin K.

Buckwheat

- DASH: Fat: ✓ Sodium: ✓ Sugar: ✓
- Diverticulitis: Stage 1: ✗ Stage 2: ✗ Stage 3: ✓
- Histamine: ✗
- Lectin: ✗
- Oxalate: ✗
- Salicylates: ✓

DASH Diet (Hypertension): Allowed. It is gluten-free, and according to Olga In The Kitchen's blog, it's just as simple to prepare as white rice. *Saturated fat content: 0.741g (per 100g), Sodium content: 1mg (per 100g) less than 1% daily value based on a 2,000 calorie diet, Sugar content: N/A (per 100g).*

Diverticulitis: No solid foods can be eaten at stage one, the clear liquids diet. Allowed on the high-fiber diet.

Histamine: Avoid.

Lectins: Lectins are present but the lectin content may be reduced by soaking, sprouting and fermenting the buckwheat (source: *Irena Macri, Nutrition Coach*).

Oxalates: Buckwheat flour, whole-groat is listed as very high (15.0mg & up) (source: *University of Chicago*). In fact they list it as one of their highest oxalate foods, though they optimistically note: *Rhubarb and spinach are so high you just cannot eat them. Rice bran is something few will miss, the same for buckwheat groats.*

Salicylates: Buckwheat is a highly nutritious whole grain that's not only gluten-free but very low in salicylates.

Butter

- DASH: Fat: ✗ Sodium: ✓ Sugar: ✓
- Diverticulitis: Stage 1: ✗ Stage 2: ✓ Stage 3: ✗
- Histamine: ✓

- Lectin: 🤐
- Oxalate: ✔
- Salicylates: ✔

Not all butter is created equal. We recommend opting for grass-fed butter because of the higher proportion of healthy fats. It's easy to find. Lots of the butter in your local supermarket will hopefully be grass-fed, organic and affordable. Grass-fed butter is also rich in Vitamin A which is necessary for normal vision, the immune system and reproduction (source: *Healthline*).

DASH Diet (Hypertension): WebMD suggests using low-fat or fat-free butter and halving your usual serving. Mayo Clinic notes "*margarine usually tops butter when it comes to heart health*". As butter comes from animal fat, there's more saturated fat. If you want to have butter, make sure it is unsalted too. *Saturated fat content: 51g (per 100g), Sodium content: 11mg (per 100g) less than 1% daily value based on a 2,000 calorie diet, Sugar content: 0.1g (per 100g).*

Diverticulitis: It's thought that butter contains no fiber. Allowed in moderation.

Histamine: Cultured butter is usually well-tolerated according to SIGHI.

Lectins: The whole subject of butter gets more complicated. Butters made with A2 milk (from cows that originate in the Channel Islands and Southern France) are possibly better for a low-lectin diet (source: *Claudia Curici, Author*). Avoid butter produced from A1 milk (regular milk with casein protein). We appreciate that it's difficult to know how shop bought milk is produced and suggest testing carefully.

Oxalates: Thought to have little or no oxalates.

Salicylates: All trustworthy lists consider butter to be very low in salicylates; however, to avoid potential ill effects that can come from hormones and additives, choose grass-fed, organic butter.

Cabbage

- DASH: Fat: ✔ Sodium: ✔ Sugar: ✔
- Diverticulitis: Stage 1: ✘ Stage 2: ✘ Stage 3: ✔
- Histamine: 🤐
- Lectin: ✔
- Oxalate: ✔
- Salicylates: ✔

DASH Diet (Hypertension): Allowed. Cabbage is thought to contain high levels of potassium which may help lower blood pressure. Eat 4-5 servings of vegetables a day. *Saturated fat content: 0g (per 100g), Sodium content: 18mg (per 100g), less than 1% daily value based on a 2,000 calorie diet, Sugar content: 3.2g (per 100g).*

Diverticulitis: No solid foods can be eaten at stage one, the clear liquids diet. Cabbage is an excellent source of fiber. Allowed on the high-fiber diet.

Histamine: We love cabbage. It's very versatile and (important one) very cheap, even organic. However, caution. Pickled cabbage is not good - the pickling makes it high-histamine.

Lectins: Falls under the cruciferous vegetable family (includes broccoli, kale, Brussel sprouts, radish etc.). These are thought to be your low-lectin friend.

Oxalates: It is thought to be very low in oxalates along with similar veggies like endive, cauliflower, and lettuce.

Salicylates: Thankfully cabbage is low in salicylates as well as being versatile and cheap, even when purchasing organic. Plus, just a half-cup cooked provides about a third of your daily vitamin C requirements.

Cactus pear

- DASH: Fat: ✓ Sodium: ✓ Sugar: ✓
- Diverticulitis: Stage 1: ✗ Stage 2: ✗ Stage 3: ✓
- Histamine: 😖
- Lectin: ✓
- Oxalate: 😖
- Salicylates: 😖

Also known as *prickly pear* and *cactus fruit*, cactus pears resemble pears in size and shape but it is not in the pear family. According to Mayo Clinic, cactus pears are promoted for treating diabetes, high cholesterol, obesity and hangovers. Enjoy as part of a healthy diet.

DASH Diet (Hypertension): Allowed and consume 4-5 servings of vegetables a day. According to Mayo Clinic, cactus pears are promoted for treating diabetes, high cholesterol, obesity and hangovers. Enjoy as part of a healthy diet. *Saturated fat content: 0.1g (per 100g), Sodium content: 5mg (per 100g) less than 1% daily value based on a 2,000 calorie diet, Sugar content: N/A (per 100g).*

Diverticulitis: No solid foods can be eaten at stage one, the clear liquids diet. Allowed on the high-fiber diet.

Histamine: Test carefully.

Lectins: It's thought that these may be eaten on a low-lectin diet.

Oxalates: Proceed with caution. Studies suggest the oxalate content of cactus pears differs depending on whether they are raw or mature.

Salicylates: There isn't a lot of information on them related to salicylates, a small clinical study published by medical analysis website eHealthMe found those who consumed it did not show an increase in salicylate levels in their bloodstream. Consume in limited amounts until you know how it will affect you. Cactus pears have a high vitamin, mineral, and antioxidant content.

Cardamom

- DASH: Fat: ✓ Sodium: ✓ Sugar: ✓
- Diverticulitis: Stage 1: ✗ Stage 2: ✗ Stage 3: ✓
- Histamine: ✓
- Lectin: 😖
- Oxalate: ✗
- Salicylates: ✗

Seeds from the cardamom plant. A number of sources outline the benefits of cardamom and even call it *"the Queen Spices"*. A study found "antibacterial and anti-inflammatory properties" of cardamom against periodontal infections (source: *Souissi M, Azelmat J, Chaieb K, Grenier D. Antibacterial and anti-inflammatory activities of cardamom (Elettaria cardamomum) extracts: Potential therapeutic benefits for periodontal infections*).

DASH Diet (Hypertension): Allowed. *Saturated fat content: 0.7g (per 100g), Sodium content: 18mg (per 100g) less than 1% daily value based on a 2,000 calorie diet, Sugar content: N/A (per 100g).*

Diverticulitis: No solid foods can be eaten at stage one, the clear liquids diet. Allowed on the high-fiber diet.

Histamine: Love cardamom so much. One of the most exotic spices. A nice way to add a little sweetness to recipes.

Lectins: Note that most seeds aren't allowed on a low-lectin diet but the health benefits of cardamom outweigh it. Test carefully.

Oxalates: Many spices are high in oxalates and cardamom appears to be one of the highest. This is from PubMed: *Spices, such as cinnamon, cloves, cardamom, garlic, ginger, cumin, coriander and turmeric are used all over the world as flavouring and colouring ingredients in Indian foods. Previous studies have shown that spices contain variable amounts of total oxalates but there are few reports of soluble oxalate contents. In this study, the total, soluble and insoluble oxalate contents of ten different spices commonly used in Indian cuisine were measured. Total oxalate content ranged from 194 (nutmeg) to 4,014 (green cardamom) mg/100 g DM, while the soluble oxalate contents ranged from 41 (nutmeg) to 3,977 (green cardamom) mg/100 g DM. Overall, the percentage of soluble oxalate content of the spices ranged from 4.7 to 99.1% of the total oxalate content which suggests that some spices present no risk to people liable to kidney stone formation, while other spices can supply significant amounts of soluble oxalates and therefore should be used in moderation.*

Salicylates: Most spices are either high or very high in salicylates. Cardamom has been listed in both categories among reliable lists, making it best avoided or used in small amounts.

Carrot

- DASH: Fat: ✓ Sodium: ✓ Sugar: ✓
- Diverticulitis: Stage 1: ✗ Stage 2: ✓ Stage 3: ✓
- Histamine: ✓
- Lectin: ✓
- Oxalate: ✗
- Salicylates: ✓

DASH Diet (Hypertension): Allowed. It's thought that eating carrots raw may be more beneficial in reducing blood pressure (source: *Healthline*). Aim for 4-5 servings of vegetables a day. *Saturated fat content: 0g (per 100g), Sodium content: 69mg (per 100g), 2% daily value based on a 2,000 calorie diet, Sugar content: 4.7g (per 100g).*

Diverticulitis: No solid foods can be eaten at stage one, the clear liquids diet. Raw carrots are high in fiber but you may eat peeled and cooked carrots on a low-fiber diet.

Histamine: More veggies on the 'good list'.

Lectins: Contain relatively little lectin.

Oxalates: Highish - one 100 g of carrot contains 15 mg of oxalates (source: *St. Joseph's Healthcare Hamilton*).

Salicylates: Fresh carrots contain a low to moderate amount of salicylates. Sources vary with some claiming there is under .25 mg per 100 g, But other sources categorize carrots as moderate in salicylates.

Cashew nut

- DASH: Fat: ✗ Sodium: ✓ Sugar: ✗
- Diverticulitis: Stage 1: ✗ Stage 2: ✗ Stage 3: ✓
- Histamine: 😐
- Lectin: ✗
- Oxalate: ✗
- Salicylates: ✓

Did you know that raw cashew nuts are toxic? This is due to a chemical called urushiol contained in the shells and this is why cashew nuts sold in stores have been roasted or steamed before shelled (source: *Medicine Net*).

DASH Diet (Hypertension): Cashew nuts are high in saturated fat and whilst the DASH diet recommends eating foods that are low in saturated fat, cashews are a source of good saturated fat which is thought to be linked to better cholesterol levels (source: *Insider*). Eat no more than 4-5 servings a week and go for unsalted nuts.

Saturated fat content: 8g (per 100g), Sodium content: 12mg (per 100g), less than 1% daily value based on a 2,000 calorie diet, Sugar content: 6g (per 100g).

Diverticulitis: No solid foods can be eaten at stage one, the clear liquids diet. Cashew nuts are rich in fiber. Allowed on the high-fiber diet.

Histamine: Medium histamine as we react and know other people who do too. Experts vary on cashew nuts. Some lists suggest they can be okay in small quantities.

Lectins: High in lectins, but cooking helps reduce lectin content. Still one to approach extremely cautiously.

Oxalates: High. Nuts like walnuts and cashews are high but thought to have slightly lower levels of oxalates than almonds; about 30 mg per ounce (source: *St. Joseph's Healthcare Hamilton*).

Salicylates: Cashews have little to no salicylates and provide important nutrients, including plant protein and heart-healthy fats.

Cassava

- DASH: Fat: ✔ Sodium: ✔ Sugar: ✔
- Diverticulitis: Stage 1: ✘ Stage 2: ✔ Stage 3: ✘
- Histamine: ✔
- Lectin: ✔
- Oxalate: 😕
- Salicylates: 😕

DASH Diet (Hypertension): Allowed. High in potassium as a cup of cassava is thought to contain 558 mg which is 16% to 21% of the daily recommendation (source: *verywellfit*). Why not have cassava on the side instead of grains? *Saturated fat content: 0.1g (per 100g), Sodium content: 14mg (per 100g), less than 1% daily value based on a 2,000 calorie diet, Sugar content: 1.7g (per 100g).*

Diverticulitis: No solid foods can be eaten at stage one, the clear liquids diet. Cassava is low in fiber so they're allowed on the low-fiber diet.

Histamine: Delicious as a flour and great gluten-free alternative.

Lectins: Cassava is thought to be fine to consume in limited quantities unless you have a pre-existing health condition. Cassava flour is also lectin-free. According to Lectin Free Mama's blog, cassava flour *"yields the fluffiest, most bread-like baked goods you can imagine"*. Why not try baking with cassava flour?

Oxalates: Delicious as a flour but is it high in oxalates? We've done lots of research on cassava as an ingredient and the lists tend to disagree and vary widely. We would suggest proceeding with caution as some think cassava contains significant amounts of oxalates. As always, it may well be an individual thing, but cassava is one we cannot rate highly.

Salicylates: While there are some reliable lists that note cassava as a low salicylate food, others advise to proceed with caution as it is believed to be high in amygdalin which can cause a reaction in some who are salicylate sensitive. Cassava is a root vegetable that is often used in flour form and that can make the salicylate content of store-bought treats high.

Cauliflower

- DASH: Fat: ✔ Sodium: ✔ Sugar: ✔
- Diverticulitis: Stage 1: ✘ Stage 2: ✘ Stage 3: ✔
- Histamine: ✔

- Lectin: ✔
- Oxalate: ✔
- Salicylates: 😕

DASH Diet (Hypertension): Allowed. Researchers found sulforaphane (the active ingredient in cauliflower) helps to reduce blood pressure (source: *OHSU Research News*). Eat 4-5 servings of vegetables a day. *Saturated fat content: 0.1g (per 100g), Sodium content: 30mg (per 100g) 1% daily value based on a 2,000 calorie diet, Sugar content: 1.9g (per 100g).*

Diverticulitis: No solid foods can be eaten at stage one, the clear liquids diet. Allowed on the high-fiber diet.

Histamine: Acceptable.

Lectins: Falls under the cruciferous vegetable family (includes broccoli, kale, cabbage, radish etc.). These are thought to be low-lectin and rich in vitamin C, folate and fiber.

Oxalates: Thought to be low in oxalates.

Salicylates: WebMD and several other reputable sites list cauliflower as having a high level of salicylates; however some rank it low or moderate. The Cauliflower salicylate content has been shown in analysis to have approximately .25 mg per 100 g, but it seems to vary. This makes it difficult to rate accurately, making it important to pay attention to how your body reacts to small amounts initially.

Celery

- DASH: Fat: ✔ Sodium: ✔ Sugar: ✔
- Diverticulitis: Stage 1: 😕 Stage 2: 😕 Stage 3: ✔
- Histamine: ✔
- Lectin: ✔
- Oxalate: ✘
- Salicylates: ✔

DASH Diet (Hypertension): Celery sticks are great as a quick, healthy snack. Just check the nutritional values of any sauce you use. Allowed and eat 4-5 servings of vegetables a day. *Saturated fat content: 0.042g (per 100g), Sodium content: 80mg (per 100g) 3% daily value based on a 2,000 calorie diet, Sugar content: 1.34 g (per 100g).*

Diverticulitis: No solid foods can be eaten at stage one, the clear liquids diet but you can juice the celery to remove some fiber content. We suggest testing carefully on the clear-liquid stage and low-fiber diet. Raw celery is high in fiber so it is allowed on the high-fiber diet.

Histamine: Some say this can be histamine-lowering.

Lectins: Good news, celery fans. Celery falls under the lowest lectin content options for a low-lectin diet.

Oxalates: High in oxalates, Listed as a 'Food to avoid' on the Unusual Ingredients website, and this verdict is borne out by many of the respected lists in our sources table above.

Salicylates: Across the board, celery is listed as being a low salicylate food and it is filled with nutrients, including vitamins A, C, and K, calcium and potassium.

Cep mushrooms

- DASH: Fat: ✘ Sodium: ✘ Sugar: ✘
- Diverticulitis: Stage 1: ✘ Stage 2: 😕 Stage 3: ✔
- Histamine: 😕

- Lectin: ✓
- Oxalate: ✓
- Salicylates: ✓

Also known as *Penny Bun*.

DASH Diet (Hypertension): The values based on the USDA's database suggests this mushroom is high in saturated fat, sodium and sugar content. Avoid. *Saturated fat content: 3.1g (per 100g), Sodium content: 304mg (per 100g), 12% daily value based on a 2,000 calorie diet, Sugar content: 32g (per 100g).*

Diverticulitis: No solid foods can be eaten at stage one, the clear liquids diet. Test cautiously on the low-fiber diet. Whilst this mushroom doesn't contain the highest amounts of fiber compared to other veg, it can still be eaten on the high-fiber diet.

Histamine: 'Shrooms massively vary from person to person and from mushroom to mushroom. Test carefully.

Lectins: Mushrooms are also thought to fall under the lowest lectin content options for a low-lectin diet.

Oxalates: See "Mushrooms"

Salicylates: See "Mushrooms"

Chamomile and chamomile tea

- DASH: Fat: ✓ Sodium: ✓ Sugar: ✓
- Diverticulitis: Stage 1: ✓ Stage 2: ✓ Stage 3: ✗
- Histamine: ✓
- Lectin: ✓
- Oxalate: ✓
- Salicylates: 😐

DASH Diet (Hypertension): Allowed. It's thought that chamomile may lower blood pressure. *Saturated fat content: 0.002g (per 100g), Sodium content: 1mg (per 100g) less than 1% daily value based on a 2,000 calorie diet, Sugar content: 0g (per 100g).*

Diverticulitis: Tea with no milk or cream is allowed at stage one, the clear liquid diet. Chamomile contains no fiber so they're allowed on the low-fiber diet.

Histamine: Acceptable.

Lectins: Tea is thought to be a better choice for a low-lectin diet than coffee. Tea is approved on a low-lectin diet.

Oxalates: Low, just 0.4-0.67 mg per cup (source: *National Library of Medicine*).

Salicylates: Herbal teas are often high in salicylates; however, chamomile has a moderately low amount according to several sites, with up to .25 mg per 100 g. Because of inconsistencies, test carefully. Depending on your body chemistry you may tolerate it when consumed in limited amounts.

Champagne

- DASH: Fat: ✓ Sodium: ✓ Sugar: ✓
- Diverticulitis: Stage 1: ✗ Stage 2: ✗ Stage 3: ✗
- Histamine: ✗
- Lectin: 😐
- Oxalate: ✓
- Salicylates: ✗

DASH Diet (Hypertension): Allowed. Drink alcohol sparingly on the DASH diet. You don't have to eliminate champagne completely although it's good to limit consumption. The University of Reading found champagne may be good for your heart and circulation by increasing the availability of nitric oxide therefore, improving the functioning of your blood vessels. *Saturated fat content: 0g (per 100g), Sodium content: 5mg (per 100g) less than 1% daily value based on a 2,000 calorie diet, Sugar content: 0.79g (per 100g).*

Diverticulitis: See alcohol.

Histamine: See comments on 'Alcohol'.

Lectins: Possibly fairly high in lectins. However, a rare treat may be okay. For example, Dr Steven Gundry permits drinking champagne occasionally. However we would not recommend making this a regular part of your low-lectin diet.

Oxalates: See alcohol.

Salicylates: Alcoholic beverages like champagne and sparkling wine are considered to be on the higher end of the scale. Unfortunately - high in salicylates. Of course, there are also the other negative health effects of alcohol to consider.

Chard

- DASH: Fat: ✓ Sodium: ✗ Sugar: ✓
- Diverticulitis: Stage 1: ✗ Stage 2: ✗ Stage 3: ✓
- Histamine: ✓
- Lectin: ✓
- Oxalate: ✗
- Salicylates: 🤔

Chard is also known by other names including *Swiss chard, Roman kale, Sicilian beet, Chilean beet, silverbeet, leaf beat, spinach beet, and mangold.*

DASH Diet (Hypertension): Chard is naturally higher in sodium than other vegetables. It's thought to contain high levels of nitrates which helps reduce blood pressure (source: *Medical News Today*). *Saturated fat content: 0.03g (per 100g), Sodium content: 213mg (per 100g), 9% daily value based on a 2,000 calorie diet, Sugar content: 1.1g (per 100g).*

Diverticulitis: No solid foods can be eaten at stage one, the clear liquids diet. Allowed on the high-fiber diet.

Histamine: Low histamine.

Lectins: Thought to be low in lectins.

Oxalates: High in oxalate. One to put in your 'avoid' list. Sally K. Norton writes, *"Just one half-cup of steamed white-stalked swiss chard has about 500 mg of oxalate and ½ cup of steamed red swiss chard has over 900 mg of oxalate. Steamed spinach has about 700 mg per ½ cup."* All of which tells you chard, swiss chard, silver beet, or whatever you want to call it, is on the avoid list on a low-oxalate diet.

Salicylates: There isn't a lot of information about chard in relation to salicylates, but some sites do list it as having a high amount besides being very high in oxalates. It may be best to avoid, or at minimum proceed with caution.

Cheddar cheese

- DASH: Fat: ✗ Sodium: ✗ Sugar: ✓
- Diverticulitis: Stage 1: ✗ Stage 2: ✓ Stage 3: ✗

- Histamine: ✗
- Lectin: ✗
- Oxalate: ✓
- Salicylates: ✓

DASH Diet (Hypertension): Low in sugar but thought to be high in saturated fat and sodium content. Avoid. *Saturated fat content: 21g (per 100g), Sodium content: 621mg (per 100g) 25% daily value based on a 2,000 calorie diet, Sugar content: 0.5g (per 100g).*

Diverticulitis: No solid foods can be eaten at stage one, the clear liquids diet. Cheddar cheese contains no fiber so they're allowed on the low-fiber diet.

Histamine: See comments on cheeses. Look for softer cheese alternatives.

Lectins: It's thought that cheddar cheese is the *"most concentrated form of casein in any food"* and given that cheeses high in casein proteins are high in lectins, avoid.

Oxalates: See "Cheeses"

Salicylates: See "Cheeses"

Cheese made from unpasteurized "raw" milk

- DASH: Fat: ✗ Sodium: ✗ Sugar: ✓
- Diverticulitis: Stage 1: ✗ Stage 2: ✓ Stage 3: ✗
- Histamine: ✗
- Lectin: 🤔
- Oxalate: ✓
- Salicylates: ✓

Raw milk cheeses include Camembert, Brie, Roquefort, Blue, Washed Rinds etc. (source: *Cheese Grotto*).

DASH Diet (Hypertension): We've based the below on raw milk cheddar cheese. Low in sugar but thought to be high in saturated fat and sodium content. *Saturated fat content: 14.3g (per 100g), Sodium content: 482mg (per 100g) 21% daily value based on a 2,000 calorie diet, Sugar content: 0g (per 100g)* (source: *Eat this much*).

Diverticulitis: No solid foods can be eaten at stage one, the clear liquids diet. Raw cheese contains no fiber so they're allowed on the low-fiber diet.

Histamine: See comments on cheeses. Look for softer cheese alternatives.

Lectins: Lectin content depends on the type of soft cheese. For example, it's thought that Brie is high in lectins. Test carefully.

Oxalates: See "Cheeses"

Salicylates: See "Cheeses"

Cheeses

- DASH: Fat: ✗ Sodium: ✗ Sugar: ✓
- Diverticulitis: Stage 1: ✗ Stage 2: ✓ Stage 3: ✗
- Histamine: Soft cheese: 🤔 Hard cheese: ✗
- Lectin: 🤔
- Oxalate: ✓
- Salicylates: ✓

DASH Diet (Hypertension): Cheese in general is thought to be low in sugar but high in saturated fat and sodium content. Check the nutritional labels for each cheese. Cleveland Clinic recommends going for naturally low-sodium cheese such as Swiss, goat, brick ricotta and fresh mozzarella. Avoid processed and hard cheeses. *Saturated fat content: 21g (per 100g), Sodium content: 621mg (per 100g) 25% daily value based on a 2,000 calorie diet, Sugar content: 0.5g (per 100g).*

Diverticulitis: No solid foods can be eaten at stage one, the clear liquids diet. Cheese contains no fiber, so they're allowed on a low-fiber diet.

Histamine: Soft cheeses tend to be much lower histamine options than hard cheeses and blue cheeses. The younger the cheese the less likely it is to be high and histamine or histamine-releasing. Again as with everything involving histamine, test extremely carefully. One batch of cheese will not be the same as another in histamine. Soft cheeses such as mozzarella ricotta and spreadable soft cheese may be tolerated. Avoid hard cheeses.

Lectins: Cheeses tend to differ. It's thought that cheeses high in casein proteins such as Cheddar, Brie, Gouda and Edam are high in lectins. Certain cheeses acquire lectins from the molds that grow within it, for example, blue cheese (source: *Understanding Arthritis, The Clinical Way Forward by W. Fox, D. Freed*). Goat and sheep cheeses are acceptable on a low-lectin diet. However, some sources suggest that consuming dairy products such as cheese increases inflammation so it should be avoided altogether. A study confirmed *"the ability of dairy products to modulate inflammatory processes in humans is an important but unresolved issue"* and *"future research should thus better combine food and nutritional sciences to adequately follow the fate of these nutrients along the gastrointestinal and metabolic axes"*. It therefore seems that more research is needed before concluding whether cheese should be avoided. Test carefully (source: *Bordoni A, Danesi F, Dardevet D, Dupont D, Fernandez AS, Gille D, Nunes Dos Santos C, Pinto P, Re R, Rémond D, Shahar DR, Vergères G. Dairy products and inflammation: A review of the clinical evidence*).

Oxalates: Most cheeses are low in oxalate or completely free of it. These include, among others; American Cheese, Cheddar Cheese, Low Fat Cheese Cottage Cheese, Low Fat Cottage Cheese, Cottage Cheese, Cream Cheese and Mozzarella Cheese and other cheeses too. This is because dairy is free of oxalate. It's also high in calcium, so it is a good choice, although cheese can have other health implications which should be carefully considered.

Salicylates: Other than blue cheeses, most cheeses are thought to be very low in salicylates. It contains high amounts of vitamins A and B-12 along with calcium, zinc, riboflavin, and phosphorus. Choose cheeses made from 100 percent grass-fed animals for the highest level of nutrients and avoid processed types which may contain salicylates along with other potentially harmful ingredients.

Cherry

- DASH: Fat: ✔ Sodium: ✔ Sugar: ✘
- Diverticulitis: Stage 1: ✘ Stage 2: ✘ Stage 3: ✔
- Histamine: 😖
- Lectin: ✔
- Oxalate: ✔
- Salicylates: ✘

DASH Diet (Hypertension): Low in saturated fat and sodium content but high in sugar. Interestingly, a study found drinking tart cherry juice lowers LDL cholesterol and total cholesterol. The study noted longer follow-up studies are needed to further assess the benefits (source: *Chai SC, Davis K, Wright RS, Kuczmarski MF, Zhang Z. Impact of tart cherry juice on systolic blood pressure and low-density lipoprotein cholesterol in older adults: a randomized controlled trial*). *Saturated fat content: 0.1g (per 100g), Sodium content: 3mg (per 100g) less than 1% daily value based on a 2,000 calorie diet, Sugar content: 8g (per 100g).*

Diverticulitis: No solid foods can be eaten at stage one, the clear liquids diet. Allowed on the high-fiber diet.

Histamine: Sometimes a debate about cherries. We buy ours frozen to lock in the nutrients and prevent any increase in histamine.

Lectins: Cherries are thought to be low lectin.

Oxalates: Low oxalate, with different lists suggesting between 3-9 mg per 100 g.

Salicylates: Sour cherries have a moderate amount of salicylates, up to .49 mg per 100 g; however, fresh sweet cherries contain a high level, up to 1 mg per 100 g. Canned sweet cherries should be avoided as they are even higher in salicylates and often contain other unwanted ingredients. Note that we have found some conflicting information, with some experts noting cherries (without indicating the type) as very high in salicylates. Based on this, avoid them altogether or choose only sour cherries, consumed in small amounts.

Chia, chia seeds

- DASH: Fat: ✗ Sodium: ✓ Sugar: ✓
- Diverticulitis: Stage 1: ✗ Stage 2: ✗ Stage 3: ✓
- Histamine: ✓
- Lectin: ✗
- Oxalate: ✗
- Salicylates: ✗

DASH Diet (Hypertension): Eat only 4-5 servings a week. Eating Well's website notes chia seeds as part of the DASH diet and a heart-healthy lifestyle. *Saturated fat content: 3.3g (per 100g), Sodium content: 16mg (per 100g), less than 1% daily value based on a 2,000 calorie diet, Sugar content: N/A (per 100g).*

Diverticulitis: No solid foods can be eaten at stage one, the clear liquids diet. Allowed on the high-fiber diet.

Histamine: Those with histamine stomach issues may want to soak a small amount of chia seeds first and eat in moderation.

Lectins: High in lectins. One to put on your 'avoid' list. Soaking the chia seeds helps reduce lectin content. Why not try basil seeds? These are basil plants' seeds that are edible and similar to chia seeds, and they become gelatinous when added to liquid. Basil seeds are a great lectin free alternative.

Oxalates: Very high, 380 mg oxalate per quarter cup of chia seeds (Source: *US National Library of Medicine*). It should be noted that you may consume a much smaller amount than a quarter cup, but the oxalate levels will still be high.

Salicylates: While there is very little information on the amount of salicylates in chia seeds, and they don't appear to have been tested in many studies, chia is a member of the mint family which contains a very high level of salicylates.

Those sensitive have reported adverse reactions to chia seeds, including ringing in the ears.

Chicken

- DASH: Fat: ✗ Sodium: ✓ Sugar: ✓
- Diverticulitis: Stage 1: ✗ Stage 2: ✓ Stage 3: ✗
- Histamine: ✓
- Lectin: ✓
- Oxalate: ✓
- Salicylates: ✓

DASH Diet (Hypertension): Remove chicken skin before eating. Chicken is often injected with saltwater solutions during processing (source: *Health Central*) to keep it juicy. Go for chicken not injected with fat or salt. Always check the nutrition labels before buying and eat no more than 2 servings a day. *Saturated fat content: 3.8g (per 100g), Sodium content: 82mg (per 100g), 3% daily value based on a 2,000 calorie diet, Sugar content: 0g (per 100g).*

Diverticulitis: No solid foods can be eaten at stage one, the clear liquids diet. Meat contains no fiber so chicken is allowed on the low-fiber diet.

Histamine: Must be organic and fresh, not leftovers. The longer food has been left to sit, the more histamine it has. Canned food, which takes many years to expire, is the worst as far as histamine content is concerned. In summary, canned chicken is terrible, organic freshly cooked chicken is great!

Lectins: Multiple sources confirm that chicken may be consumed on a low-lectin diet. Avoid corn-fed chicken and opt for pasture-raised chicken.

Oxalates: Very low as long as it's organic and fresh.

Salicylates: Chicken contains no or only trace amounts of salicylates, provided it is not processed, such as smoked and cured meats. Choose fresh, organic options.

Chickpeas

- DASH: Fat: ✓ Sodium: ✓ Sugar: ✗
- Diverticulitis: Stage 1: ✗ Stage 2: ✗ Stage 3: ✓
- Histamine: ✗
- Lectin: ✗
- Oxalate: 😐
- Salicylates: ✓

DASH Diet (Hypertension): Low in saturated fat and sodium content but high in sugar. Eat in moderation. Mayo Clinic notes chickpeas as a healthy option on the DASH diet. *Saturated fat content: 0.6g (per 100g), Sodium content: 24mg (per 100g), 1% daily value based on a 2,000 calorie diet, Sugar content: 11g (per 100g).*

Diverticulitis: No solid foods can be eaten at stage one, the clear liquids diet. Allowed on the high-fiber diet.

Histamine: We react particularly badly to chickpeas, and while that's just a personal opinion, the general vibe seems to be - avoid them.

Lectins: High in lectins. One to put on your 'avoid' list.

Oxalates: Thought to be low to medium in oxalate. Sources vary between 5-10mg per cup.

Salicylates: Chickpeas are not only low in salicylates, but these legumes are also an excellent source of fiber, iron, potassium, selenium, magnesium, and B vitamins to support heart health.

Chicory

- DASH: Fat: ✓ Sodium: ✓ Sugar: ✓
- Diverticulitis: Stage 1: ✗ Stage 2: ✗ Stage 3: ✓
- Histamine: ✓
- Lectin: ✓
- Oxalate: ✗
- Salicylates: ✗

Also known as endive. This lovely veg is great for balancing flavors in dishes as it adds acidity and sweetness (source: *Mashed*).

DASH Diet (Hypertension): Allowed. Eat 4-5 servings of vegetables a day.

Diverticulitis: No solid foods can be eaten at stage one, the clear liquids diet. The fiber is found in the root. Chicory root is often used as a fiber supplement added to processed food (source: *Eat This*).

Histamine: Acceptable.

Lectins: Thought to be low lectin.

Oxalates: Some debate. Many consider it quite high in oxalates, with 21 mg per 100g (*Agriculture Handbook No. 8-11, Vegetables and Vegetable Products, 1984*).

Salicylates: Avoid chicory as all our sources and lists rank it very high in salicylates.

Chili pepper, red, fresh

- DASH: Fat: ✓ Sodium: ✓ Sugar: ✓
- Diverticulitis: Stage 1: ✗ Stage 2: 😕 Stage 3: ✓
- Histamine: ✗
- Lectin: ✗
- Oxalate: 😕
- Salicylates: ✗

DASH Diet (Hypertension): Capsaicin is the compound in chilis that gives heat. Research has shown that this compound reduces blood pressure in rats, but it hasn't yet been carried out on humans (source: *Nicswell*). Allowed on the DASH diet. *Saturated fat content: 0g (per 100g), Sodium content: 9mg (per 100g) less than 1% daily value based on a 2,000 calorie diet, Sugar content: 5g (per 100g).*

Diverticulitis: No solid foods can be eaten at stage one, the clear liquids diet. Whilst chili peppers don't contain the highest amounts of fiber compared to other veg, they can still be eaten on a high-fiber diet. Test carefully on a low-fiber diet.

Histamine: Spicy foods can release histamine, which becomes an issue when added to the histamine produced by seasonal allergies or histamine intolerance. You could try to avoid spicy food when your histamine symptoms are acting up.

Lectins: High in lectins. One to put on your 'avoid' list. They are a part of the nightshade family, which is high in lectins, particularly in the seeds and peels.
To reduce lectin content, Precision Nutrition recommends peeling and de-seed chili peppers before cooking. This is because the highest concentration of lectins can be found in the seeds of plants (source: *Diagnosis Diet*).

Oxalates: Hot chili peppers are thought to be moderate in oxalates. Red peppers are low.

Salicylates: Hot chili peppers are very high in salicylates, although the capsaicin they contain may reduce adverse effects. Consume minimally until you know how your body will react. Avoid sweet peppers which contain a high level of salicylates without the capsaicin.

Chives

- DASH: Fat: ✓ Sodium: ✓ Sugar: ✓
- Diverticulitis: Stage 1: ✗ Stage 2: ✗ Stage 3: ✓
- Histamine: 😕

- Lectin: ✔
- Oxalate: ✔
- Salicylates: ✔

DASH Diet (Hypertension): Allowed. *Saturated fat content: 0.1g (per 100g), Sodium content: 3mg (per 100g), less than 1% daily value based on a 2,000 calorie diet, Sugar content: 1.9g (per 100g).*

Diverticulitis: No solid foods can be eaten at stage one, the clear liquids diet. Allowed on the high-fiber diet.

Histamine: Test carefully.

Lectins: Thought to be low lectin.

Oxalates: Low oxalate with less than 5mg per serving. (source: *Urinary Stones website*). As we've emphasized throughout this book, proceed with caution as the more you look into this area, the more debate there is. The Agriculture Handbook No. 8-11, Vegetables and Vegetable Products, 1984 lists chives as high oxalate, so proceed with caution. The Heal With Food website notes; *Like parsley, chives are only used in small amounts in cooking. Therefore, chives are not likely to contribute much oxalic acid to your diet, although they are among the most concentrated dietary sources of oxalates. A 100-serving of chives is estimated to provide 1480 milligrams of oxalates.*

Salicylates: Chives are low in salicylates while being nutrient dense. They include the carotenoids lutein and zeaxanthin to support eye health and reduce the risk of macular degeneration.

Chocolate

- DASH: Fat: ✘ Sodium: ✔ Sugar: ✘
- Diverticulitis: Stage 1: ✘ Stage 2: ✔ Stage 3: ✔
- Histamine: ✘
- Lectin: ✔
- Oxalate: ✘
- Salicylates: 😖

Due to the sugar content in chocolate, we recommend 85-90% cocoa solids as these contain little sugar.

DASH Diet (Hypertension): Dark chocolate is high in flavonoids which can help lower bad cholesterol (source: *heart.org*). The American Medical Association has published a study which shows eating dark chocolate can lower blood pressure however, Alice H. Lichtenstein, the Gershoff professor of nutrition science and policy at Tufts University in Boston states: *"While dark chocolate has more flavanols than other types of chocolate, the data to suggest there is enough to have a health effect is thin at this point."* Be aware of caffeine in chocolate as this may cause a spike in blood pressure. Avoid white chocolate as it's high in saturated fat and sugar. It's also not considered chocolate since it's not made of cocoa solids.

Diverticulitis: No solid foods can be eaten at stage one, the clear liquids diet. Allowed on the low-fiber diet. Go for dark chocolate on the high-fiber diet.

Histamine: Chocolate is considered a histamine liberator rather than high in histamine. This is clearly not good news. White chocolate can be tolerated a little better, but frustratingly many seem to react to that too. All this applies to chocolate drinks, mousses, sauces, anything cacao related and so on.

Lectins: Chocolate is made from fermented cocoa beans. A study found the fermentation process reduces lower lectin content (source: *Sá AGA, Moreno YMF, Carciofi BAM. Food processing for the improvement of plant proteins digestibility*). Chocolate contains lectins, but these aren't 'toxic lectins', which means the lectins present do not harm the gut barrier (source: *Paleo in the UK*).

Oxalates: Chocolate is potentially high in oxalates. This from Science Direct: *As chocolate is considered as a high oxalate food (Williams and Wilson, 1990, Massey et al., 1993, Noonan and Savage, 1999, Mendonça et al., 2003), The*

Oxalosis & Hyperoxaluria Foundation (OHF, 2004) recommends that affected persons should avoid eating chocolate. Note that white chocolate may be better tolerated on a low oxalate diet.

Salicylates: Chocolate has been reported by some with sensitivity to salicylates to have an adverse effect. However, many reputable sites consider dark chocolate not made with raw sugar to have a low amount, with reports that it is well-tolerated.

Cilantro

- DASH: Fat: ✓ Sodium: ✓ Sugar: ✓
- Diverticulitis: Stage 1: 🤐 Stage 2: ✓ Stage 3: ✗
- Histamine: 🤐
- Lectin: ✓
- Oxalate: ✓
- Salicylates: ✗

Also known as *coriander*. Cilantro comes from the coriander plant.

DASH Diet (Hypertension): Allowed. Saturated fat content: 0.014g (per 100g), Sodium content: 46mg (per 100g) 2% daily value based on a 2,000 calorie diet, Sugar content: 0.87g (per 100g).

Diverticulitis: Cilantro leaves aren't allowed, but you may add cilantro herb mix to broths for more flavor. Allowed on the low-fiber diet.

Histamine: Test carefully.

Lectins: Thought to be low-lectin.

Oxalates: Low oxalate (source: *Urinary Stones website*). They (specifically) note that this relates to 9 raw sprigs.

Salicylates: There is conflicting information about how much salicylates it contains, although most reliable sources categorize it as "high", making it best to avoid or limit to very small amounts.

Cinnamon

- DASH: Fat: ✓ Sodium: ✓ Sugar: ✓
- Diverticulitis: Stage 1: ✗ Stage 2: 🤐 Stage 3: ✓
- Histamine: 🤐
- Lectin: ✓
- Oxalate: ✗
- Salicylates: ✗

DASH Diet (Hypertension): Allowed. A study found consuming cinnamon short term is linked to a reduction in systolic blood pressure and diastolic blood pressure (source: *Akilen R, Pimlott Z, Tsiami A, Robinson N. Effect of short-term administration of cinnamon on blood pressure in patients with prediabetes and type 2 diabetes*.) Saturated fat content: 0.3g (per 100g), Sodium content: 10mg (per 100g), less than 1% daily value based on a 2,000 calorie diet, Sugar content: 2.2g (per 100g).

Diverticulitis: No solid foods can be eaten at stage one, the clear liquids diet. Allowed on the high-fiber diet. Test cautiously on the low-fiber diet.

Histamine: This is one of those where the major food lists seem to disagree. Some say cinnamon is low histamine, and some say it is high. From personal experience, we have noted a reaction to histamine. Hence, we suggest acting cautiously as reactions vary from person to person.

Lectins: Acceptable.

Oxalates: High oxalate as per several studies. This is from PubMed on spices: *Spices, such as cinnamon, cloves, cardamom, garlic, ginger, cumin, coriander and turmeric are used all over the world as flavoring and coloring ingredients in Indian foods. Previous studies have shown that spices contain variable amounts of total oxalates but there are few reports of soluble oxalate contents. In this study, the total, soluble and insoluble oxalate contents of ten different spices commonly used in Indian cuisine were measured. Total oxalate content ranged from 194 (nutmeg) to 4,014 (green cardamom) mg/100 g DM, while the soluble oxalate contents ranged from 41 (nutmeg) to 3,977 (green cardamom) mg/100 g DM. Overall, the percentage of soluble oxalate content of the spices ranged from 4.7 to 99.1% of the total oxalate content which suggests that some spices present no risk to people liable to kidney stone formation, while other spices can supply significant amounts of soluble oxalates and therefore should be used in moderation.*

Salicylates: As with many spices, cinnamon is high in salicylates with at least 1 mg per 100 g.

Citrus fruits

- DASH: Fat: ✓ Sodium: ✓ Sugar: ✓
- Diverticulitis: Stage 1: ✗ Stage 2: ✗ Stage 3: ✓
- Histamine: ✗
- Lectin: 😐
- Oxalate: 😐
- Salicylates: 😐

DASH Diet (Hypertension): Allowed. Citrus fruits contain vitamins and minerals and may lower your blood pressure. **Lemon**: *Saturated fat content: 0g (per 100g), Sodium content: 2mg (per 100g), less than 1% daily value based on a 2,000 calorie diet, Sugar content: 2.5g (per 100g).* **Lime**: *Saturated fat content: 0g (per 100g), Sodium content: 2mg (per 100g), less than 1% daily value based on a 2,000 calorie diet, Sugar content: 1.7g (per 100g).*

Diverticulitis: Citrus juices are allowed only if strained, and no seeds and pulp. They're an excellent source of fiber, so you may have them on a high-fiber diet.

Histamine: Most citrus seems to be very high in histamine.

Lectins: These include lemons, limes and oranges, which are thought to contain some lectins to varying degrees. The opinion is split with oranges. One source confirmed oranges are a source of lectins. However, another source noted oranges contain D-Mannose, a powerful natural lectin-blocker. The lectin content varies depending on the fruit, but as citrus fruits are high in antioxidants, the benefits outweigh the negatives. It's thought that these could be enjoyed in moderation.

Oxalates: Varies. For example, oranges are very high, and lemons are low. Check individual foods.

Salicylates: See the individual fruit as it varies depending on the type of citrus fruit. For example, lemons and limes are low or medium in salicylates; however, oranges are very high.

Clover

- DASH: No information
- Diverticulitis: Stage 1: ✗ Stage 2: ✗ Stage 3: ✓
- Histamine: ✗
- Lectin: ✗
- Oxalate: ✗
- Salicylates: 😐

A part of the pea family.

Diverticulitis: No solid foods can be eaten at stage one, the clear liquids diet. Allowed on the high-fiber diet.

Histamine: Avoid.

Lectins: A study found a pea lectin gene in the roots of white clover (*source: Sugar-Binding Activity of Pea Lectin Expressed in White Clover Hairy Roots by Clara L. Díaz, Trudy J. J. Logman, Hanneke C. Stam and Jan W. Kijne*). Best to avoid.

Oxalates: Very high, contains oxalic acid, which depletes the body of calcium and iron. Red clover is toxic.

Salicylates: While there is not much information on clover related to its salicylate content, some reliable sites list it as low in salicylates. This refers to clover, which can be red or white. The blossoms of red clover contain salicylates, but we could not find an analysis of the amount. That makes this wild veggie difficult to rate, so once again, we ask you to proceed with caution. Edible clover is a wild vegetable that's said to be highly nutritious though it's often referred to as a "weed." As clover is a foraged food, if you choose to consume it, be sure that it is gathered from a pristine, clean source that has not been treated with chemicals.

Cloves

- DASH: Fat: ✗ Sodium: ✗ Sugar: ✓
- Diverticulitis: Stage 1: ✗ Stage 2: ✗ Stage 3: ✓
- Histamine: ✓
- Lectin: ✓
- Oxalate: ✗
- Salicylates: ✗

DASH Diet (Hypertension): Low in sugar but thought to be high in saturated fat and sodium content. Avoid. *Saturated fat content: 5.438g (per 100g), Sodium content: 243mg (per 100g) 11% daily value based on a 2,000 calorie diet, Sugar content: 2.38g (per 100g)* (source: *Fatsecret Platform API*).

Diverticulitis: No solid foods can be eaten at stage one, the clear liquids diet. Allowed on the high-fiber diet.

Histamine: Low histamine.

Lectins: Thought to be allowed on a low-lectin diet (source: *Daytona Wellness Center*).

Oxalates: Very high in oxalate. Thought to be one of the highest oxalate-containing spices.

Salicylates: Cloves have ranked anywhere from high to extremely high in salicylates.

Cocoa butter and cacao butter

- DASH: Fat: ✗ Sodium: ✓ Sugar: ✓
- Diverticulitis: Stage 1: ✗ Stage 2: ✓ Stage 3: ✗
- Histamine: ✗
- Lectin: ✓
- Oxalate: ✗
- Salicylates: 😷

DASH Diet (Hypertension): Cocoa has been found to reduce blood pressure however, "*long-term trials are needed to determine whether cocoa has an effect on cardiovascular events.*" (source: *Ried K, Fakler P, Stocks NP. Effect of cocoa on blood pressure. Cochrane Database Syst Rev. 2017;4(4):CD008893*). *Saturated fat content: 60g (per 100g), Sodium content: 0mg (per 100g), Sugar content: 0mg (per 100g).*

Diverticulitis: Contains no fiber, so allowed on the low-fiber diet.

Histamine: Histamine-releasing. See our comments on 'Chocolate'.

Lectins: Cocoa butter is the fat extracted from the cocoa bean. Thought to be low-lectin. As chocolate can be high in sugar, we recommend 85-90% cocoa solids as these are lower sugar and may represent a healthier choice.

Oxalates: High oxalate. Note the below from PubMed: *Cocoa is a strong carrier of oxalic acid (average: 400 mg per 100 g). In three calcium oxalate stone formers clinical observation had suggested excessive intake of cocoa products contributing to calculus formation.*

Salicylates: Chocolate, cocoa and cacao butters are thought to have low-to-moderate salicylates and are generally safe, including cocoa/cacao butter. The information is not definitive, however, and therefore, test carefully.

Cocoa drinks, powder, etc

- DASH: Fat: ✘ Sodium: ✘ Sugar: ✓
- Diverticulitis: Stage 1: ✘ Stage 2: 😐 Stage 3: ✓
- Histamine: ✘
- Lectin: ✓
- Oxalate: ✘
- Salicylates: ✘

As chocolate can be high in sugar, we recommend 85-90% cocoa solids as these are lower sugar and may represent a healthier choice.

DASH Diet (Hypertension): Low in sugar but thought to be high in saturated fat and sodium content. Avoid. *Saturated fat content: 8g (per 100g), Sodium content: 21mg (per 100g) less than 1% daily value based on a 2,000 calorie diet, Sugar content: 1.8g (per 100g).*

Diverticulitis: Test cocoa powder carefully on a low-fiber diet. Allowed on the high-fiber diet.

Histamine: See 'Chocolate'.

Lectins: Thought to be low-lectin.

Oxalates: High oxalate. Note the following from Heal With Food: *A 2011 study published in the Journal of Food Composition and Analysis found that the total oxalate content of cocoa powder can range from 650 to 783 milligrams per 100 grams on a dry matter basis (cocoa powder contains very little moisture which implies the values would be very similar on a wet weight basis).*

Salicylates: See "Chocolate"

Coconut and coconut derivatives

- DASH: Fat: ✘ Sodium: ✓ Sugar: ✘
- Diverticulitis: Stage 1: ✘ Stage 2: 😐 Stage 3: ✓
- Histamine: 😐
- Lectin: ✓
- Oxalate: ✓
- Salicylates: ✘

DASH Diet (Hypertension): High in saturated fat and sugar. Avoid cooking with coconut oil. There has been little research done to support the benefits of coconut oil however, we know that drinking coconut water decreases blood pressure (source: *Alleyne T, Roache S, Thomas C, Shirley A. The control of hypertension by use of coconut water and mauby: two tropical food drinks. West Indian Med J. 2005*). Saturated fat content: 30g (per 100g), Sodium content: 20mg (per 100g) less than 1% daily value based on a 2,000 calorie diet, Sugar content: 6g (per 100g).

Diverticulitis: No solid foods can be eaten at stage one, the clear liquids diet. Coconut oil and coconut water are allowed on a low-fiber diet. Coconut, in general, is allowed on the high-fiber diet.

Histamine: Some aspects of coconut can be high in histamine, particularly coconut aminos. In addition, while most people seem to be okay with coconut, there are a significant number of histamine intolerant people who do not get on well with it, so test carefully. Coconut milk sometimes has several additives in them, so they go from being low histamine to high histamine and say that it's something to look out for on the ingredients label.

Lectins: Thought to be low-lectin.

Oxalates: Low in oxalates according to several sources.

Salicylates: Fresh coconut, dried coconut (also referred to as desiccated), coconut milk and coconut water contain a moderate amount of salicylates, up to .49 mg per 100 g. Coconut oil, on the other hand, is thought to be very high in salicylates, with over 1 mg per 100 g.

Coffee

- DASH: Fat: ✓ Sodium: ✓ Sugar: ✓
- Diverticulitis: Stage 1: ✓ Stage 2: 😕 Stage 3: ✓
- Histamine: 😕
- Lectin: 😕
- Oxalate: ✓
- Salicylates: 😕

DASH Diet (Hypertension): Allowed. Go for Americano to reduce your calorie intake. Coffee lovers: don't drink too much, as over four cups a day may increase your blood pressure (source: *NHS*). *Saturated fat content: 0g (per 100g), Sodium content: 2mg (per 100g), less than 1% daily value based on a 2,000 calorie diet, Sugar content: 0g (per 100g).*

Diverticulitis: Only allowed with no milk or cream. It seems that the cream or milk normally causes flare-ups in coffee rather than the coffee itself. Decaffeinated coffee is allowed on a low-fiber diet. Coffee contains higher amounts of soluble fiber than other drinks, so it is allowed on the high-fiber diet.

Histamine: Oh, this is something we could write an entire book about. Coffee massively divides people in the histamine intolerance community. About half of us seem to tolerate it, and half don't. That seems to be a benefit of seeking low histamine, low mold, organic, and low toxin coffees.

Lectins: Coffee is important! But it is one of those ingredients where opinion is split. Some of our research has shown coffee contains lectins, but as these aren't 'toxic lectins', the lectins present in coffee don't harm the gut barrier, so it's ok to consume. Others believe raw coffee beans are high in lectins, but since the beans are heated, drinking coffee is safe. And then there is yet more opinion, including a school of thought which suggests coffee should be avoided altogether. So who to believe? The major lists disagree considerably, and you should test carefully. This is one reason we wrote this book, so we could reflect on all the different points of view for you, and you can make your own mind up.

Oxalates: Low oxalate. Thank goodness for that!

Salicylates: We know you want good information on coffee and salicylates - the news is mixed! Decaf coffee contains negligible amounts of salicylates; however, regular coffee is considered to have a moderate level that ranges from .10 mg to .64 mg per 100 g depending on the brand. If you must have a hot drink, coffee is better than most teas but to limit salicylates, go without the caffeine or mix half decaf and half regular.

Coriander

See *cilantro*.

Cornflakes

- DASH: Fat: ✓ Sodium: ✗ Sugar: ✗
- Diverticulitis: Stage 1: ✗ Stage 2: ✓ Stage 3: ✗
- Histamine: ✓
- Lectin: ✗
- Oxalate: ✓
- Salicylates: ✓

DASH Diet (Hypertension): Avoid. Cornflakes may increase your risk of developing heart disease (source: *Health Day*). *Saturated fat content: 0.1g (per 100g), Sodium content: 729mg (per 100g), 30% daily value based on a 2,000 calorie diet, Sugar content: 10g (per 100g).*

Diverticulitis: No solid foods can be eaten at stage one, the clear liquids diet. Allowed on the low-fiber diet.

Histamine: Several foods might be well-tolerated in terms of histamine intolerance but will not be particularly good for your overall health. Let's put cornflakes into that category. They should be low in histamine as long as they don't have additives. But there are healthier breakfast options.

Lectins: High in lectins. One to put on your 'avoid' list.

Oxalates: Several foods might be well-tolerated in terms of oxalates but will not be good for your overall health. Let's put cornflakes into that category. Online specialist The Kidney Dietitian notes; *Rice Chex, Rice Krispies, cornflakes and Cheerios are very low oxalate cereal choices…. Some cold cereals are very high in oxalate – be careful to avoid bran flakes (yes, that includes Raisin Bran), rice bran and shredded wheat. These all have more than 25 grams of oxalate per 100 g.*

Salicylates: Ready-to-eat cereals are low in salicylates, including cornflakes; however, they aren't the healthiest option, and other ingredients may well change the salicylate content.

Courgette

- DASH: Fat: ✓ Sodium: ✓ Sugar: ✓
- Diverticulitis: Stage 1: ✗ Stage 2: 😶 Stage 3: ✓
- Histamine: ✓
- Lectin: ✗
- Oxalate: ✓
- Salicylates: ✗

Also known as *zucchini*.

DASH Diet (Hypertension): Allowed. You may use courgette as a base to make a healthy Bruschetta. *Saturated fat content: 0.1g (per 100g), Sodium content: 8mg (per 100g), less than 1% daily value based on a 2,000 calorie diet, Sugar content: 2.5g (per 100g).*

Diverticulitis: No solid foods can be eaten at stage one, the clear liquids diet. Allowed on the high-fiber diet but peel the skin on the low-fiber diet.

Histamine: Acceptable.

Lectins: Mixed opinion. Some sources say these are high in lectin, whereas some say it's ok to consume.

Oxalates: Thought to have less than 2 mg of oxalate per serving.

Salicylates: There isn't much information about courgette and salicylates; however, some sources include it in the "high" or "very high" categories. Therefore, we advise avoiding dishes or consuming only small amounts.

Crab

- DASH: Fat: ✓ Sodium: ✗ Sugar: ✓
- Diverticulitis: Stage 1: ✗ Stage 2: ✓ Stage 3: ✗
- Histamine: ✗
- Lectin: ✓
- Oxalate: ✓
- Salicylates: ✓

Crab shells contain high levels of glucosamine (a natural compound found in cartilage)? In fact, glucosamine supplements are often made from lobster, shrimps, crabs and crawfish shells. Next time, don't throw the shells away. Grind them up and sprinkle them over food (source: *Human Food Bar*).

DASH Diet (Hypertension): High in sodium, best to avoid. Whilst crab is high in sodium, we came across sources that suggest the benefits outweigh the risks. Crabs are high in protein and low in calories. Mayo Clinic's website features crab cakes as a sample menu created by the clinic's dieticians. *Saturated fat content: 0.1g (per 100g), Sodium content: 1,072mg (per 100g), 44% daily value based on a 2,000 calorie diet, Sugar content: 0g (per 100g).*

Diverticulitis: No solid foods can be eaten at stage one, the clear liquids diet. Allowed on the low-fiber diet.

Histamine: See comments elsewhere on fish and seafood.

Lectins: Thought to be low-lectin.

Oxalates: Low.

Salicylates: Provided it's fresh and has not been preserved with sulfites, crab contains no or very little salicylates. It's packed with high levels of vitamin B12, selenium, and omega-3 fatty acids.

Cranberries and cranberry juice

- DASH: Fat: ✓ Sodium: ✓ Sugar: ✗
- Diverticulitis: Stage 1: ✓ Stage 2: ✗ Stage 3: ✓
- Histamine: ✓
- Lectin: ✓
- Oxalate: ✓
- Salicylates: ✗

DASH Diet (Hypertension): Despite cranberry juice being high in sugar, they're full of vitamins and minerals. Cranberries are thought to boost your digestive health and promote heart health (source: *heart.org*). A study found cranberry juice reduced blood pressure and lipoprotein profile. However, further studies are needed to verify the findings (source: *Richter CK, Skulas-Ray AC, Gaugler TL, Meily S, Petersen KS, Kris-Etherton PM. Effects of Cranberry Juice Supplementation on Cardiovascular Disease Risk Factors in Adults with Elevated Blood Pressure: A Randomized Controlled Trial. Nutrients. 2021 Jul 29;13(8):2618.*) Avoid dried cranberries as they're full of sugar.
Cranberries: *Saturated fat content: 0.1g (per 100g), Sodium content: 3mg (per 100g) less than 1% daily value based on a 2,000 calorie diet, Sugar content: 65g (per 100g).* **Cranberry juice**: *,Saturated fat content: 0g (per 100g), Sodium content: 2mg (per 100g), less than 1% daily value based on a 2,000 calorie diet, Sugar content: 12g (per 100g).*

Diverticulitis: Allowed only if cranberry juice is clear with no seeds and pulp. Cranberry is allowed on the high-fiber diet.

Histamine: Tolerated.

Lectins: We recommend cranberries on a low lectin diet. It's a great option and may help lower your lectin levels. Health Canal's website refers to cranberry as a *"natural lectin blocker"* as it binds lectins and helps the body absorb them more efficiently.

Oxalates: 0.1 - 2.9 mg very low (source: *Low Oxalate Diet - Mark O'Brien MD*).

Salicylates: Cranberries, whether the fruit, juice or canned in a sauce, are high in salicylates with at least 1 mg per 100 g.

Crawfish

- DASH: Fat: ✓ Sodium: ✓ Sugar: ✓
- Diverticulitis: Stage 1: ✗ Stage 2: ✓ Stage 3: ✗
- Histamine: ✗
- Lectin: ✗
- Oxalate: ✓
- Salicylates: ✓

Also known as *crayfish*.

DASH Diet (Hypertension): Allowed. *Saturated fat content: 0.163g (per 100g), Sodium content: 62mg (per 100g) 3% daily value based on a 2,000 calorie diet, Sugar content: 0g (per 100g).*

Diverticulitis: No solid foods can be eaten at stage one, the clear liquids diet. Seafood contains no fiber, so crawfish is allowed on the low-fiber diet.

Histamine: Fish are generally not tolerated well.

Lectins: Avoid crayfish as lectins have been found in freshwater crayfish (source: *Zhang XW, Wang XW, Sun C, Zhao XF, Wang JX. C-type lectin from red swamp crayfish Procambarus clarkii participates in cellular immune response.*)

Oxalates: Likely to be low oxalate.

Salicylates: Fish contains no to only trace amounts of salicylates, according to most reliable sources.

Crayfish

- DASH: Fat: ✓ Sodium: ✓ Sugar: ✓
- Diverticulitis: Stage 1: ✗ Stage 2: ✓ Stage 3: ✗
- Histamine: ✗
- Lectin: ✗
- Oxalate: ✓
- Salicylates: ✓
- Also known as *crawfish*.

DASH Diet (Hypertension): Allowed. *Saturated fat content: 0.163g (per 100g), Sodium content: 62mg (per 100g), 3% daily value based on a 2,000 calorie diet, Sugar content: 0g (per 100g)* (source: *Fatsecret Platform API*).

Diverticulitis: No solid foods can be eaten at stage one, the clear liquids diet. Seafood contains no fiber, so crayfish are allowed on a low-fiber diet.

Histamine: Fish are generally not tolerated well.

Lectins: Avoid crayfish as lectins have been found in freshwater crayfish (source: *Zhang XW, Wang XW, Sun C, Zhao XF, Wang JX. C-type lectin from red swamp crayfish Procambarus clarkii participates in cellular immune response.*)

Oxalates: Likely to be low oxalate.

Salicylates: Fish contains no to only trace amounts of salicylates, according to most reliable sources.

Cream cheeses

- DASH: Fat: ✗ Sodium: ✗ Sugar: ✓
- Diverticulitis: Stage 1: ✗ Stage 2: ✗ Stage 3: ✓
- Histamine: 😖
- Lectin: 😖
- Oxalate: ✓
- Salicylates: ✓

DASH Diet (Hypertension): Low in sugar but thought to be high in saturated fat and sodium content. It's also high in calories. Avoid. If you want to enjoy cheese, go for naturally low-sodium cheese such as swiss, goat, brick ricotta and fresh mozzarella. *Saturated fat content: 19g (per 100g), Sodium content: 321mg (per 100g), 13% daily value based on a 2,000 calorie diet, Sugar content: 3.2g (per 100g).*

Diverticulitis: No solid foods can be eaten at stage one, the clear liquids diet. Cheese contains no fiber, so they're allowed on a low-fiber diet.

Histamine: See other comments on cheese. Organic is best.

Lectins: Some sources claim that very high-fat dairy products such as cream cheeses are low in casein and therefore low in lectin. Other sources mention all dairy products contain casein and should be avoided. Test carefully.

Oxalates: Fine. See "Cream" below or "Cheeses" above.

Salicylates: See "Cheeses" or "Cream"

Cream

- DASH: Fat: ✗ Sodium: ✓ Sugar: ✓
- Diverticulitis: Stage 1: ✗ Stage 2: ✓ Stage 3: ✗
- Histamine: ✓
- Lectin: 😖
- Oxalate: ✓
- Salicylates: ✓

DASH Diet (Hypertension): Avoid cream, but if you eat it, go for low-fat cream and consume it in moderation. Too much saturated fat is linked to poor heart health. *Saturated fat content: 12g (per 100g), Sodium content: 40mg (per 100g), 1% daily value based on a 2,000 calorie diet, Sugar content: 0.1g (per 100g).*

Diverticulitis: Cream contains no fiber, so they're allowed on the low-fiber diet.

Histamine: Aim for grass-fed. If fermented, histamine levels rise.

Lectins: As above, some sources claim that very high-fat dairy products such as cream are low in casein and therefore low in lectin. Other sources mention all dairy products contain casein and should be avoided. Test carefully.

Oxalates: Fine. The University of Virginia Digestive Health Center notes: *Eat plenty of calcium-rich foods. Calcium binds to oxalate so that it isn't absorbed into your blood and cannot reach your kidneys. Dairy is free of oxalate and high in calcium, so it is an ideal choice. Choose skim, low fat, or full-fat versions depending on your weight goals. If you are lactose intolerant, look for lactose free dairy such as Lactaid brand, or eat yogurt or kefir instead.*

Salicylates: Creams of all types are very low in salicylates, provided the ingredient list does not include additives. It's high in calcium but also high in fat, meaning it should be consumed in small amounts. Generally, an organic grass-fed heavy cream is the better choice as it contains nutrients like antioxidants and healthy fats.

Cress

- DASH: Fat: ✓ Sodium: ✓ Sugar: ✓
- Diverticulitis: Stage 1: 😐 Stage 2: ✗ Stage 3: ✓
- Histamine: 😐
- Lectin: 😐
- Oxalate: ✗
- Salicylates: ✗

DASH Diet (Hypertension): A great garnish and allowed on the DASH diet. They're full of nitrates which help lower your blood pressure. *Saturated fat content: 0g (per 100g), Sodium content: 14mg (per 100g), less than 1% daily value based on a 2,000 calorie diet, Sugar content: 4.4g (per 100g).*

Diverticulitis: Eating raw cress isn't allowed, but you may add cress herb mix to broths for more flavor. Allowed on the high-fiber diet.

Histamine: Test carefully.

Lectins: Thought to contain some lectins. Test carefully.

Oxalates: Cress naturally contains extremely high amounts of oxalates. It's recommended that people who are at risk of experiencing urinary lithiasis absolutely reduce their intake of oxalate-rich foods like cress. They should not consume cress at all.

Salicylates: One of the oldest leafy greens known to humans, there is limited information on the amount of salicylates in cress. Watercress contains .49 to 1 mg, considered a "high" level, which is why we feel it's best to avoid or consume in small amounts until you know how it will affect you.

Cucumber

- DASH: Fat: ✓ Sodium: ✓ Sugar: ✓
- Diverticulitis: Stage 1: 😐 Stage 2: 😐 Stage 3: ✓
- Histamine: ✓
- Lectin: 😐
- Oxalate: ✓
- Salicylates: ✗

DASH Diet (Hypertension): Allowed, plus they're low in calories too. There are so many ways to include cucumber in your diet. You can eat them raw with salad or as a snack. They can be cooked or used for smoothies. Eat 4-5 servings of vegetables a day. *Saturated fat content: 0.034g (per 100g), Sodium content: 2mg (per 100g) less than 1% daily value based on a 2,000 calorie diet, Sugar content: 1.67g (per 100g).*

Diverticulitis: Clear cucumber juice is allowed. No solid foods can be eaten at stage one, the clear liquids diet. Peel the skin and do not eat the seeds on a low-fiber diet. Whilst cucumber doesn't contain the highest amounts of fiber compared to other veg, it can still be eaten on the high-fiber diet.

Histamine: Note - this is fresh cucumber, not pickled. Anything pickled is a different story.

Lectins: Mixed opinion. Precision Nutrition recommends peeling and deseeding cucumbers before cooking to reduce lectin content. This is because the highest concentration of lectins can be found in the seeds of plants (source: *Diagnosis Diet*). However, Kimberly Gomer, Director of Nutrition at the Pritikin Longevity Center in Miami confirmed the lectins found in cucumber "*whether cooked or consumed raw, do not appear to cause significant GI problems*". Test carefully.

Oxalates: Thought to be low in oxalate.

Salicylates: Most reliable sources categorize cucumber as high in salicylates, with analysis sometimes showing it to have .78 mg per 100 g.

Cumin

- DASH: Fat: ✗ Sodium: ✗ Sugar: ✓
- Diverticulitis: Stage 1: ✗ Stage 2: ✗ Stage 3: ✓
- Histamine: ✗
- Lectin: ✓
- Oxalate: ✗
- Salicylates: ✗

DASH Diet (Hypertension): Low in sugar but thought to be high in saturated fat and sodium content. The National Kidney Foundation's website lists cumin as allowed on this diet. Harvard Medical School's website suggests making a vegetarian chili with cumin and other ingredients such as beans, onions, canned tomatoes, minced garlic and chili powder. *Saturated fat content: 1.5g (per 100g), Sodium content: 168 mg (per 100g), 7% daily value based on a 2,000 calorie diet, Sugar content: 2.3g (per 100g).*

Diverticulitis: Allowed on the high-fiber diet.

Histamine: The big lists seem to divert quite considerably around cumin. We love using it in our cooking and would hate to give it up and seem to react okay. However, not everybody agrees that cumin is a suitable ingredient for those with histamine intolerance.

Lectins: After careful analysis, we've found limited research on cumin and lectins. Since dill is a part of the Apiaceae family (which includes parsley, parsnip, celery and carrot), cumin could be allowed on a low-lectin diet.

Oxalates: Cumin seed is potentially one of the higher oxalate foods. Looking for an alternative? Online specialist Sally K. Norton has some brilliant suggestions. She says; *Try the curry styles of Thailand. Instead of cumin and turmeric (Indian style curry ingredients), Thai food is seasoned with various combinations of the following: cayenne, chili peppers, garlic, lime, lemongrass, mint, coconut milk, fish sauce, onion, and cilantro.*

Salicylates: This is very much on our 'avoid list'. Cumin seed contains a very high level of salicylates. According to NutritionFacts.org, eating a teaspoon of it is like taking baby aspirin (one of the highest salicylate products you can eat).

Curry

- DASH: Fat: ✗ Sodium: ✓ Sugar: ✓
- Diverticulitis: Stage 1: ✗ Stage 2: ✗ Stage 3: ✓
- Histamine: 🤔
- Lectin: ✓
- Oxalate: 🤔
- Salicylates: ✗

DASH Diet (Hypertension): Curries are usually made of turmeric, coriander, cumin, ginger, chili powder and pepper. WebMD noted a study that found *"people who eat more curry powder are less likely to have high blood pressure"*. Why not try chickpea curry? Eating Well's website features a quick and healthy recipe. *Saturated fat content: 2.2g (per 100g), Sodium content: 52mg (per 100g), 2% daily value based on a 2,000 calorie diet, Sugar content: 2.8g (per 100g).*

Diverticulitis: No solid foods can be eaten at stage one, the clear liquids diet. Allowed on the high-fiber diet.

Histamine: Clearly not all curries are created equal: Curry leaves are thought to be low in histamine, but curry powder is high in histamine. In addition, you want to check for the level of spice and additives.

Lectins: Depends on the ingredients in the curry. The most common ingredients are thought to include garlic, ginger, turmeric, black pepper and onions, to name a few, which are allowed on a low-lectin diet.

Oxalates: Check for ingredients and the level of spice and additives. This is from PubMed: *Spices, such as cinnamon, cloves, cardamom, garlic, ginger, cumin, coriander and turmeric are used all over the world as flavoring and coloring ingredients in Indian foods. Previous studies have shown that spices contain variable amounts of total oxalates but there are few reports of soluble oxalate contents. In this study, the total, soluble and insoluble oxalate contents of ten different spices commonly used in Indian cuisine were measured. Total oxalate content ranged from 194 (nutmeg) to 4,014 (green cardamom) mg/100 g DM, while the soluble oxalate contents ranged from 41 (nutmeg) to 3,977 (green cardamom) mg/100 g DM. Overall, the percentage of soluble oxalate content of the spices ranged from 4.7 to 99.1% of the total oxalate content which suggests that some spices present no risk to people liable to kidney stone formation, while other spices can supply significant amounts of soluble oxalates and therefore should be used in moderation.*

Salicylates: Curry is a popular Indian dish with a sauce seasoned with spices like turmeric, cumin, ginger, coriander, and chili pepper. While ingredients may vary, as all recipes typically call for many spices that are very high in salicylates, it is best avoided. Live Strong notes: *Herbs and spices suspected to have high amounts of salicylates include curry, cumin powder, dill, oregano, hot paprika, rosemary, thyme, turmeric and vegemite. Many of which are found in curries (but not vegemite!)*

Dates

- DASH: Fat: ✓ Sodium: ✓ Sugar: ✗
- Diverticulitis: Stage 1: ✗ Stage 2: ✗ Stage 3: ✓
- Histamine: 🤔
- Lectin: 🤔
- Oxalate: ✗
- Salicylates: ✗

DASH Diet (Hypertension): Low in saturated fat and sodium content but high in sugar. The sugar in dates is natural, and several sources suggest dates are allowed on the DASH diet. *Saturated fat content: 0.032g (per 100g), Sodium content: 0mg (per 100g), Sugar content: 63.35g (per 100g)* (source: Fatsecret Platform API).

Diverticulitis: No solid foods can be eaten at stage one, the clear liquids diet. Allowed on the high-fiber diet.

Histamine: Experts disagree on whether dates are high or low histamine. Test carefully.

Lectins: Moderate lectin content. Test carefully.

Oxalates: They are high in oxalates with 24 mg per date, according to the University of Chicago. They're also very high in sugar.

Salicylates: Dates are high in natural sugars and are said to contain a very high amount of salicylates. Avoid. Note: Dried apricots and dates are often considered among the highest salicylate foods.

Dextrose

- DASH: Fat: ✓ Sodium: ✓ Sugar: ✗
- Diverticulitis: Stage 1: ✓ Stage 2: ✗ Stage 3: ✓
- Histamine: ✓
- Lectin: ✗
- Oxalate: ✓
- Salicylates: ✓

Sugar from corn. There isn't any benefit from eating sugar.

DASH Diet (Hypertension): The American Heart Association recommends no more than 24g of sugar for women and no more than 36g per day for men. 100g of dextrose exceeds the sugar recommendations per day. Avoid.

Diverticulitis: As dextrose is a type of sugar and sugar is allowed on the clear liquid diet. It is also high in fiber. Dextrose is technically allowed on the clear liquid and high-fiber diet, but we suggest avoiding it as sugar isn't good for your health.

Histamine: Tolerated.

Lectins: We know that all corn foods should be avoided. Opt for honey as an alternative to sugar.

Oxalates: See "Sugar"

Salicylates: See "Sugar"

Dill

- DASH: Fat: ✓ Sodium: ✓ Sugar: ✓
- Diverticulitis: Stage 1: 😐 Stage 2: 😐 Stage 3: ✓
- Histamine: 😐
- Lectin: ✓
- Oxalate: ✓
- Salicylates: ✗

Dill is a fragrant spice that's great for freshening up your dishes.

DASH Diet (Hypertension): Allowed. *Saturated fat content: 0.1g (per 100g), Sodium content: 61mg (per 100g) 2% daily value based on a 2,000 calorie diet, Sugar content: N/A (per 100g).*

Diverticulitis: Whilst dill doesn't contain the highest amounts of fiber compared to other herbs, it can still be eaten on the high-fiber diet. Test carefully on a low-fiber diet.

Histamine: Test carefully.

Lectins: Since dill is a part of the Apiaceae family (which includes parsley, parsnip, celery and carrot), dill could be allowed on a low-lectin diet.

Oxalates: Low oxalate according to UPMC.

Salicylates: An herb in the celery family, dill is extremely high in salicylates.

Dragon fruit

- DASH: Fat: ✓ Sodium: ✓ Sugar: ✗
- Diverticulitis: Stage 1: ✗ Stage 2: ✗ Stage 3: ✓
- Histamine: ✓

- Lectin: 🤔
- Oxalate: ✗
- Salicylates: ✗

Often known as white-fleshed pitahaya. Dragon fruits are an excellent source of fiber, magnesium, iron, vitamin C, carotenoids and lycopene.

DASH Diet (Hypertension): Low in saturated fat and sodium content but high in sugar. Eat in moderation. *Saturated fat content: N/A (1 fruit), Sodium content: N/A (1 fruit), Sugar content: 8g (1 fruit).*

Diverticulitis: No solid foods can be eaten at stage one, the clear liquids diet. An excellent source of fiber. Allowed on the high-fiber diet.

Histamine: Tolerated.

Lectins: It seems that this fruit may be enjoyed as part of a healthy diet. Test carefully.

Oxalates: High, 97.1 mg/100 g (source: *Journal of Food Composition and Analysis*).

Salicylates: High in salicylates according to research published in the International Archives of Allergy and Immunology.

Dried fruit

- DASH: Fat: ✓ Sodium: ✗ Sugar: ✗
- Diverticulitis: Stage 1: ✗ Stage 2: ✗ Stage 3: ✓
- Histamine: ✓
- Lectin: 🤔
- Oxalate: 🤔
- Salicylates: ✗

These included raisins, dates, prunes, apricots, to name a few. Dried fruits are a great snack but watch the calorie and sugar content. The drying process removes water from the fruit, which means a higher sugar concentration (source: *New York Times*).

DASH Diet (Hypertension): Best to avoid, although we recommend you check the nutritional values for each dried fruit. Dates are thought to be the healthier dried fruit. See Dates above. *Saturated fat content: 0.7g (per 100g), Sodium content: 403mg (per 100g), 16% daily value based on a 2,000 calorie diet, Sugar content: 58g (per 100g).*

Diverticulitis: No solid foods can be eaten at stage one, the clear liquids diet. Dried fruits are high in fiber but are high in sugar content too, best to limit.

Histamine: Allowed on the low-histamine diet.

Lectins: We think the lectin content depends on the type of dried fruit, but it's unclear whether the drying process reduces lectin content. Test carefully.

Oxalates: Often low in oxalate. Watch out for pineapple and fig. Portion size can be a big issue. The University of Chicago notes: *Dried fruits have to be a worry because the water is taken out, so a 'portion' of dried fruit can be gigantic in oxalate content. Figs, pineapple and prunes are standouts. Just think: 1/2 cup of dried pineapple is 30 mg – not a lot of fruit for a lot of oxalate.* Elsewhere, canned pineapple is considered very high in oxalate, but canned cherries are moderate, and canned pears and peaches have little to no oxalate.

Salicylates: Dried fruits such as apricots, raisins, and prunes contain high levels of salicylates.

Dried meat

- DASH: Fat: ✗ Sodium: ✗ Sugar: ✓
- Diverticulitis: Stage 1: ✗ Stage 2: ✓ Stage 3: ✗
- Histamine: ✗
- Lectin: ✓
- Oxalate: ✓
- Salicylates: 😐

DASH Diet (Hypertension): Low in sugar but thought to be high in saturated fat and sodium content. Dried meat is a highly processed food. Avoid. *Saturated fat content: 1.6g (per 100g), Sodium content: 950mg (per 100g), 39% daily value based on a 2,000 calorie diet, Sugar content: 0g (per 100g).*

Diverticulitis: No solid foods can be eaten at stage one, the clear liquids diet. Dried meats contain no fiber, so they're allowed on the low-fiber diet.

Histamine: Unfortunately, normally very high in histamine.

Lectins: Includes grass-fed jerky, which is allowed on a low-lectin diet. Ensure these are grass-fed.

Oxalates: Should be low in oxalates.

Salicylates: Dried meat unprocessed with no seasonings contain minimal or no salicylates; however, products like beef jerky typically contain additives and spices that make it high in salicylates. This especially applies to store-bought products with a longer shelf-life and, therefore, more potential salicylate-containing additives.

Dry-cured meats

- DASH:
  - Beef: Fat: ✓ Sodium: ✗ Sugar: ✓
  - Pork: Fat: ✓ Sodium: ✗ Sugar: ✗
- Diverticulitis: Stage 1: ✗ Stage 2: ✓ Stage 3: ✗
- Histamine: ✗
- Lectin: ✓
- Oxalate: ✓
- Salicylates: 😐

These are meats that have been salted, dried and aged to preserve them from harmful bacteria. Dry-cured meats include jamon, prosciutto and salami, etc.

DASH Diet (Hypertension): They contain unhealthy amounts of sodium. Avoid. **Beef**: *Saturated fat content: 0.95g (per 100g), Sodium content: 2,790mg (per 100g), 121% daily value based on a 2,000 calorie diet, Sugar content: 2.45g (per 100g).* **Pork**: *Saturated fat content: 1g (per 100g), Sodium content: 320mg (per 100g), 14% daily value based on a 2,000 calorie diet, Sugar content: 10g (per 100g).*

Diverticulitis: No solid foods can be eaten at stage one, the clear liquids diet. Dried cured meats contain no fiber, so they're allowed on the low-fiber diet.

Histamine: Old and cured - that means high in histamine.

Lectins: As meats are generally low in lectins, dry-cured meats are allowed on a low-lectin diet. Ensure these are grass-fed.

Oxalates: Should be low in oxalates.

Salicylates: Curing uses ingredients like sugar, salt, nitrate and/or nitrite for preservation, color, and flavor. We've found it hard to get specific, accurate information that we can reliably pass on about dry-cured meats. However, given the ingredients and curing process varies, we believe that this alone makes it best treated with caution.

Duck

- DASH: Fat: ✗ Sodium: ✓ Sugar: ✓
- Diverticulitis: Stage 1: ✗ Stage 2: ✓ Stage 3: ✗
- Histamine: ✓
- Lectin: ✓
- Oxalate: ✓
- Salicylates: ✓

DASH Diet (Hypertension): Do not eat the skin and avoid crispy duck. SF Gate recommends going for baked, roasted or braised duck. Limit to one serving a day without the skin. *Saturated fat content: 10g (per 100g), Sodium content: 59mg (per 100g), 2% daily value based on a 2,000 calorie diet, Sugar content: 0g (per 100g).*

Diverticulitis: No solid foods can be eaten at stage one, the clear liquids diet. Meat contains no fiber, so duck is allowed on a low-fiber diet.

Histamine: Tolerated.

Lectins: Allowed. Opt for pasture-raised duck.

Oxalates: See "Meat"

Salicylates: See "Meat"

Egg white

- DASH: Fat: ✓ Sodium: ✗ Sugar: ✓
- Diverticulitis: Stage 1: ✗ Stage 2: ✓ Stage 3: ✗
- Histamine: 😶
- Lectin: 😶
- Oxalate: ✓
- Salicylates: ✓

DASH Diet (Hypertension): Eggs are high in cholesterol, so limit consumption (source: *Harvard Medical School*) however, a study found eggs have no significant effect on blood pressure (source: *Kolahdouz-Mohammadi R, Malekahmadi M, Clayton ZS, et al. Effect of Egg Consumption on Blood Pressure: a Systematic Review and Meta-analysis of Randomized Clinical Trials.*) *Saturated fat content: 0g (per 100g), Sodium content: 166mg (per 100g), 6% daily value based on a 2,000 calorie diet, Sugar content: 0.7g (per 100g).*

Diverticulitis: No solid foods can be eaten at stage one, the clear liquids diet. Allowed on the low-fiber diet.

Histamine: Cooked eggs without other ingredients can often be okay. Some believe that egg white can be mast cell activating. However, The Histamine Intolerance Awareness Site notes; "*The theory, that egg white is a histamine releaser has been dismissed.*" Many tolerate eggs and especially egg yolks. Always buy organic and pasture-raised.

Lectins: Depends on the type of egg. Always buy pasture-raised eggs as these contain the least amount of lectins. According to Lectin Free Mama's blog, "*duck eggs make fluffier, higher-raised baking goods than chicken eggs*". Why not try baking with duck eggs?

Oxalates: Eggs are thought to be very low/no oxalate. However, moderation may be important if you are worried about kidney stones. The Harvard Health website notes; *Limit animal protein: Eating too much animal protein, such as red meat, poultry, eggs, and seafood, boosts the level of uric acid and could lead to kidney stones.4 Oct 2013* .

Salicylates: Both egg white and yolk are salicylate free; however, according to research published in Food Additives & Contaminants: *Residues of salicylic acid in tissues and eggs may occur after drug administration or exposure of animals to feed material with high salicylate content.* The residue was found in very low concentrations with researchers noting that the eggs did not pose any risk to consumers sensitive to salicylates. Still, we consider it important to buy organic, pasture-raised eggs which contain more nutrients, including omega-3 fatty acids, beta-carotene, and vitamins A, E, and D with less saturated fat and cholesterol.

Egg yolk

- DASH: Fat: ✗ Sodium: ✓ Sugar: ✓
- Diverticulitis: Stage 1: ✗ Stage 2: ✓ Stage 3: ✗
- Histamine: 😐
- Lectin: 😐
- Oxalate: ✓
- Salicylates: ✓

DASH Diet (Hypertension): Limit egg yolk intake to no more than four a week as eggs are high in cholesterol (source: *Harvard Medical School*). Saturated fat content: 10g (per 100g), Sodium content: 48mg (per 100g), 2% daily value based on a 2,000 calorie diet, Sugar content: 0.6g (per 100g).

Diverticulitis: No solid foods can be eaten at stage one, the clear liquids diet. Allowed on the low-fiber diet.

Histamine: See comments above.

Lectins: Depends on the type of egg. Always buy pasture-raised eggs as these contain the least amount of lectins.

Oxalates: See comments above.

Salicylates: See comments above.

Elderflower cordial

- DASH: Fat: ✓ Sodium: ✓ Sugar: ✗
- Diverticulitis: Stage 1: ✓ Stage 2: ✓ Stage 3: ✗
- Histamine: ✓
- Lectin: ✗
- Oxalate: ✗
- Salicylates: ✗

DASH Diet (Hypertension): Low in saturated fat and sodium content but high in sugar. A study on mice found elderflower lowered systolic blood pressure by five percent and diastolic blood pressure by two and a half percent. More research is needed to back this up (source: *Smart Supplements Guide*). Saturated fat content: 0g (per 25ml), Sodium content: N/A (per 25ml), Sugar content: 5.6g (per 25ml).

Diverticulitis: Thought to contain very little fiber.

Histamine: Tolerated.

Lectins: Elderflower contains lectins, and it's thought to come from the same tree as elderberries. A study found lectins present in the barks of elderberries (source: *Nsimba-Lubaki M, Peumans WJ. Seasonal Fluctuations of Lectins in Barks of Elderberry (Sambucus nigra) and Black Locust (Robinia pseudoacacia)*). Test carefully.

Oxalates: High. While elderberry fruits are a good source of minerals and antioxidants, the presence of oxalates and other anti-nutrients may limit their utilization.

Salicylates: Very high in salicylates, elderflower cordial is a soft drink made with the European elder's flowers, typically combined with a solution of water and refined sugar.

Endive

- DASH: Fat: ✓ Sodium: ✓ Sugar: ✓
- Diverticulitis: Stage 1: ✗ Stage 2: ✗ Stage 3: ✓
- Histamine: ✓
- Lectin: ✓
- Oxalate: ✓
- Salicylates: ✗

DASH Diet (Hypertension): Allowed. Endive is low in calories and helps regulate blood sugar levels. It's high in potassium which is great for your heart health. *Saturated fat content: 0g (per 100g), Sodium content: 22mg (per 100g), less than 1% daily value based on a 2,000 calorie diet, Sugar content: 0.3g (per 100g).*

Diverticulitis: No solid foods can be eaten at stage one, the clear liquids diet. Allowed on the high-fiber diet.

Histamine: Tolerated.

Lectins: Acceptable on a low-lectin diet.

Oxalates: Thought to be low in oxalates.

Salicylates: Our research shows that endive is very high in salicylates.

Espresso

- DASH: Fat: ✓ Sodium: ✓ Sugar: ✓
- Diverticulitis: Stage 1: ✓ Stage 2: 😐 Stage 3: ✓
- Histamine: 😐
- Lectin: 😐
- Oxalate: ✓
- Salicylates: 😐

DASH Diet (Hypertension): Allowed. Espresso is thought to contain more caffeine than coffee. Watch out for your caffeine intake. Drinking over four cups a day may increase your blood pressure (source: *NHS*). *Saturated fat content: 0.1g (per 100g), Sodium content: 14mg (per 100g), less than 1% daily value based on a 2,000 calorie diet, Sugar content: 0g (per 100g).*

Diverticulitis: Decaffeinated coffee is allowed on the low-fiber diet. Coffee contains higher amounts of soluble fiber than other drinks, so it is allowed on the high-fiber diet.

Histamine: We've given espresso its own slot in our food list, as it's better tolerated than regular coffee, according to SIGHI. We're not sure, but they know what they are talking about. Test carefully.

Lectins: Coffee is one of those where opinion is split. Some say coffee contains lectins, but as these aren't 'toxic lectins', the lectins present in coffee don't harm the gut barrier, so it's ok to consume. Others say raw coffee beans are high in lectins, but since the beans are heated, drinking coffee is safe. Some argue that coffee should be avoided altogether. Test carefully.

Oxalates: See "Coffee"

Salicylates: See "Coffee"

Fennel

- DASH: Fat: ✔ Sodium: ✔ Sugar: ✔
- Diverticulitis: Stage 1: ✘ Stage 2: ✘ Stage 3: ✔
- Histamine: ✔
- Lectin: ✔
- Oxalate: ✘
- Salicylates: ✔

DASH Diet (Hypertension): Allowed. Fennel contains nitrates which are thought to help lower blood pressure. Eat 4-5 servings of vegetables a day. *Saturated fat content: 0.2g (per 100g), Sodium content: 52mg (per 100g), 2% daily value based on a 2,000 calorie diet, Sugar content: N/A (per 100g).*

Diverticulitis: No solid foods can be eaten at stage one, the clear liquids diet. Allowed on the high-fiber diet.

Histamine: Tolerated.

Lectins: Tolerated.

Oxalates: High, 129 mg per 10 grams (source: *Journal of Food Processing and Preservation*).

Salicylates: While the bulb of the fennel plant has a very low salicylate content, the leafy top is high in salicylates. Stick to the bulb with a fresh licorice flavor and crisp texture similar to celery, caramelizing as it cooks for a sweeter taste.

Fenugreek

- DASH: Fat: ✘ Sodium: ✔ Sugar: ✔
- Diverticulitis: Stage 1: ✘ Stage 2: ✘ Stage 3: ✔
- Histamine: ✘
- Lectin: 🫘
- Oxalate: ✘
- Salicylates: ✘

A herb that has many health benefits, such as reducing the risk of cancer, diabetes, obesity, high blood pressure and inflammation, to name a few (source: *Medical News Today*).

DASH Diet (Hypertension): Fenugreek is thought to lower blood pressure and blood sugar. A source suggests not consuming fenugreek every day. *Saturated fat content: 1.5g (per 100g), Sodium content: 0mg (per 100g), Sugar content: N/A (per 100g).*

Diverticulitis: A rich source of fiber. Allowed on the high-fiber diet.

Histamine: Avoid.

Lectins: Lectins are present in fenugreek (source: *Food and Nutrition Journal*). Test carefully.

Oxalates: According to a study, leafy vegetables such as curry, drumstick, shepu, fenugreek, coriander, radish, and onion stalks contain only insoluble oxalate, which ranges from 209.0 +/- 5.0 mg/100 g dry matter to 2,774.9 +/-18.4 mg/100 g dry matter (source: *Journal of Food Processing and Preservation*).

Salicylates: Dried fenugreek contains a high level of salicylates with at least 1 mg per 100 g, according to Molecular Nutrition & Food Research.

Feta cheese

- DASH: Fat: ✘ Sodium: ✘ Sugar: ✔

- Diverticulitis: Stage 1: ✗ Stage 2: ✓ Stage 3: ✗
- Histamine: 😕
- Lectin: 😕
- Oxalate: ✓
- Salicylates: ✓

DASH Diet (Hypertension): Low in sugar but thought to be high in saturated fat and sodium content. Limit cheese intake if you're following the DASH diet but if you must eat cheese, go for low-fat cheese such as feta. *Saturated fat content: 15g (per 100g), Sodium content: 1,116mg (per 100g), 46% daily value based on a 2,000 calorie diet, Sugar content: 4.1g (per 100g).*

Diverticulitis: No solid foods can be eaten at stage one, the clear liquids diet. Cheese contains no fiber, so they're allowed on a low-fiber diet.

Histamine: For many, feta cheese falls into the soft cheese category and is slightly better tolerated than many hard or blue-veined kinds of cheese. Again this is a matter of considerable variance between different people. It is confusing to have histamine intolerance when one person will react so badly to a particular Cheese and another won't. We totally get this, and that is why we ask you to test carefully.

Lectins: Thought to be low-lectin if made with sheep or goat's milk. Traditional feta cheese is made with sheep or goat's milk, but cow's milk is used nowadays. Check before consuming.

Oxalates: Thought to be low oxalate. See 'cheeses'.

Salicylates: Most cheeses are thought to be very low in salicylates. Choose cheeses made from 100 percent grass-fed animals for the highest level of nutrients and avoid processed types that may contain salicylates and other potentially harmful ingredients. Feta is also a lower-histamine cheese, so a good option for those with multiple intolerances.

Figs (fresh or dried)

- DASH: Fat: ✓ Sodium: ✓ Sugar: ✗
- Diverticulitis: Stage 1: ✗ Stage 2: ✗ Stage 3: ✓
- Histamine: 😕
- Lectin: ✓
- Oxalate: 😕
- Salicylates: 😕

DASH Diet (Hypertension): Low in saturated fat and sodium content but high in sugar. Eat in moderation. *Saturated fat content: 0.06g (per 100g), Sodium content: 1mg (per 100g), less than 1% daily value based on a 2,000 calorie diet, Sugar content: 16.26g (per 100g).*

Diverticulitis: No solid foods can be eaten at stage one, the clear liquids diet. Three to five figs provide approximately five grams of dirty fiber (source: *Valley Fig*). Allowed on the high-fiber diet.

Histamine: Fresh are likely to be lower histamine than dry.

Lectins: These are actually flowers and not fruit! Thought to be low-lectin.

Oxalates: See previous comments on figs and dried fruit. Dried figs sometimes have less than 5 mg of oxalate content per fig (source: *University of Chicago*). However, portion size is important. It may be a suitable alternative to dates that are high in fiber, potassium, iron, and calcium.

Salicylates: Fresh figs are low in salicylates with no more than .49 mg per 100 g; however, as with other dried fruits (see "Dried Fruits"), dried figs contain a high amount of salicylates. While most people eat dried figs, give the fresh version a go. It has a soft, jammy texture and is rich in vitamin A.

Fish

- DASH: Fat: ✗ Sodium: ✓ Sugar: ✓
- Diverticulitis: Stage 1: ✗ Stage 2: ✓ Stage 3: ✗
- Histamine: ✗
- Lectin: 😬
- Oxalate: ✓
- Salicylates: ✓

DASH Diet (Hypertension): Avoid salted fish. Fresh fish is acceptable. If the fish is canned or frozen, ensure it is low in sodium, as salt is often added to preserve the fish for longer. The DASH Diet (Hypertension) for Hypertension by Mark Jenkins and Thomas J. Moore suggests all fish are naturally low in saturated fat. They recommend choosing fish over chicken or beef. *Saturated fat content: 2.5g (per 100g), Sodium content: 61mg (per 100g) 2% daily value based on a 2,000 calorie diet, Sugar content: N/A (per 100g).*

Diverticulitis: No solid foods can be eaten at stage one, the clear liquids diet. Seafood contains no fiber, so fish is allowed on the low-fiber diet.

Histamine: All fish except freshly caught and frozen we list as high histamine. Fish also increases in histamine extraordinarily quickly. Certain fish, especially salmon, is okay if caught fresh and frozen quickly after catching. Fish freshly caught within an hour or frozen within an hour may well be better tolerated. Any fish in fishmongers or smoked should be avoided.

Lectins: Depends on the type. Check individual fish in this list. Whitefish are lobsters and are thought to be low in lectins. Avoid crayfish as lectins in freshwater crayfish (source: *Zhang XW, Wang XW, Sun C, Zhao XF, Wang JX. C-type lectin from red swamp crayfish Procambarus clarkii participates in cellular immune response*). Lectins were also reported in trout (source: *Ng TB, Fai Cheung RC, Wing Ng CC, Fang EF, Wong JH. A review of fish lectins*).

Oxalates: Likely to be low oxalate. In addition, you may like to seek fish with higher calcium levels, sardines with bones, whitebait, salmon and so on.

Salicylates: Fish contains no to only trace amounts of salicylates, according to most reliable sources.

Flaxseed (linseed)

- DASH: Fat: ✗ Sodium: ✓ Sugar: ✓
- Diverticulitis: Stage 1: ✗ Stage 2: ✗ Stage 3: ✓
- Histamine: ✓
- Lectin: ✓
- Oxalate: 😬
- Salicylates: ✗

DASH Diet (Hypertension): Eat no more than 4-5 servings a week. Eating Well's website notes flaxseeds as part of the DASH diet and a heart-healthy lifestyle. *Saturated fat content: 3.7g (per 100g), Sodium content: 30mg (per 100g) 1% daily value based on a 2,000 calorie diet, Sugar content: 1.6g (per 100g).*

Diverticulitis: No solid foods can be eaten at stage one, the clear liquids diet. High in fiber. Allowed on the high-fiber diet.

Histamine: Sprouted flaxseed is often even better tolerated than normal - but it costs more to buy.

Lectins: Tolerated on a low-lectin diet.

Oxalates: This is in the low- to moderate-oxalate group of foods, containing between 2 and 10 mg oxalate per 100 grams (source: *UPMC*).

Salicylates: We couldn't find original research on salicylate levels in flaxseed that satisfied us to include in this dictionary. Interestingly, some dermatologists treating patients with eczema have listed it as containing a moderate level and do not recommend it to those who are sensitive to salicylates. We have rated it accordingly.

Fructose (fruit sugar)

- DASH: Fat: ✔ Sodium: ✔ Sugar: ✘
- Diverticulitis: Stage 1: ✔ Stage 2: ✔ Stage 3: ✘
- Histamine: ✔
- Lectin: ✘
- Oxalate: 😉
- Salicylates: ✘

Fructose is a fruit sugar that's often used in processed foods. According to the RDH (Registered Dental Hygienists), there is no biological need for fructose. RDH lists the negative health implications of consuming fructose, such as the increased risk of obesity and type 2 diabetes to name a few.

DASH Diet (Hypertension): Because of the potential negative health implications, we recommend avoiding processed fructose where possible.

Diverticulitis: As fructose is a type of sugar, it is thought to contain no fiber.

Histamine: It might be low histamine, but you want to avoid too much sugar.

Lectins: It's unclear whether fructose contains lectins but avoid processed fructose where possible. However, foods naturally high in fructose, such as apples, pears and honey, are allowed on a low lectin diet. These may be consumed in moderation.

Oxalates: A study published in Pubmed revealed that increased fructose intake correspondingly increased the risk of forming kidney stones. It was postulated that fructose consumption increased urinary oxalate, a risk factor for calcium oxalate kidney stone disease. However, the subjects in the study did not demonstrate any changes in the excretions of oxalate, calcium, and uric acid.

Salicylates: We advise against consuming them. Additionally, the peer-reviewed journal Alternative Medicine Review reports it has caused chronic diarrhoea and/or other bowel problems in some besides contributing to obesity and diabetes. We have struggled to source trustworthy information specifically available on fructose and salicylates; therefore we cannot provide a definitive rating.

Game (meat)

- DASH: Fat: ✔ Sodium: ✔ Sugar: ✔
- Diverticulitis: Stage 1: ✘ Stage 2: ✔ Stage 3: ✘
- Histamine: ✔
- Lectin: ✔
- Oxalate: ✔
- Salicylates: ✔

DASH Diet (Hypertension): The DASH diet recommends lean meat if you have to eat meat. Game is lean, which means it's high in protein and low in fat. Allowed on the DASH diet. Eat no more than 2 servings a day. *Saturated fat content: 1g (per 100g), Sodium content: 51mg (per 100g), 2% daily value based on a 2,000 calorie diet, Sugar content: 0g (per 100g)* (source: *Nutrition Value*).

Diverticulitis: No solid foods can be eaten at stage one, the clear liquids diet. Meat contains no fiber, so game is allowed on the low-fiber diet.

Histamine: Organic meat is best.

Lectins: Tolerated. Opt for pasture-raised game.

Oxalates: Low. However, eating large portions might increase the risk of kidney stones.

Salicylates: Fresh meat, including game, contains no salicylates. Avoid cured meats.

Garlic

- DASH: Fat: ✔ Sodium: ✔ Sugar: ✔
- Diverticulitis: Stage 1: ✘ Stage 2: 😖 Stage 3: ✘
- Histamine: 😖
- Lectin: ✔
- Oxalate: ✔
- Salicylates: ✔

DASH Diet (Hypertension): Allowed. PubMed has published a study confirming garlic helps reduce blood pressure (source: *Ried K, Frank OR, Stocks NP, Fakler P, Sullivan T. Effect of garlic on blood pressure: a systematic review and meta-analysis. BMC Cardiovasc Disord*). *Saturated fat content: 0.089g (per 100g), Sodium content: 17mg (per 100g) 1% daily value based on a 2,000 calorie diet, Sugar content: 1g (per 100g)* (source: *Fatsecret Platform API*).

Diverticulitis: No solid foods can be eaten at stage one, the clear liquids diet. Garlic contains little fiber, test cautiously on the low-fiber diet.

Histamine: Garlic is relatively well tolerated, although not 100% by everybody.

Lectins: Garlic falls under the lowest lectin content options for a low-lectin diet.

Oxalates: See "Broad-leaved garlic"

Salicylates: See "Broad-leaved garlic"

Ginger

- DASH: Fat: ✔ Sodium: ✔ Sugar: ✔
- Diverticulitis: Stage 1: ✘ Stage 2: 😖 Stage 3: ✘
- Histamine: ✔
- Lectin: ✔
- Oxalate: ✘
- Salicylates: ✘

DASH Diet (Hypertension): Allowed. Ginger has been shown to reduce blood pressure. Add this spice to brighten up your dish. *Saturated fat content: 0.2g (per 100g), Sodium content: 13mg (per 100g), less than 1% daily value based on a 2,000 calorie diet, Sugar content: 1.7g (per 100g)*.

Diverticulitis: No solid foods can be eaten at stage one, the clear liquids diet. Ginger contains little fiber, test cautiously on the low-fiber diet.

Histamine: Tolerated.

Lectins: Acceptable.

Oxalates: Contains an extensive amount of total oxalate (201-4014 mg/100 g) (source: *Journal of Plant Foods for Human Nutrition*).

Salicylates: Ginger in any form, fresh, powder, or otherwise, contains a high level of salicylates with well over 1 mg per 100 g, according to our best resources.

Goat's milk

- DASH: Fat: ✗ Sodium: ✓ Sugar: ✓
- Diverticulitis: Stage 1: ✗ Stage 2: ✓ Stage 3: ✗
- Histamine: ✓
- Lectin: ✓
- Oxalate: ✓
- Salicylates: ✓

DASH Diet (Hypertension): A study found goat's milk lowers blood pressure and prevents hypertension in sedentary women. This is a great alternative to cow's milk as goat's milk is thought to be naturally lower in cholesterol. Go for low-fat goat's milk (source: *https://www.atlantis-press.com/proceedings/phico-16/25875903*). *Saturated fat content: 2.7g (per 100g), Sodium content: 50mg (per 100g), 2% daily value based on a 2,000 calorie diet, Sugar content: 4.5g (per 100g).*

Diverticulitis: Avoid at stage one the clear liquid diet as milk causes flare-ups. All liquids should be clear. Allowed on the low-fiber diet.

Histamine: Allowed.

Lectins: Goat's milk contains much less/no A1 beta-casein protein than cow's milk which means they are allowed on a low-lectin diet.

Oxalates: See "Milk"

Salicylates: See "Milk"

Goji berry

- DASH: Fat: ✓ Sodium: ✗ Sugar: ✗
- Diverticulitis: Stage 1: ✗ Stage 2: ✗ Stage 3: ✓
- Histamine: ✓
- Lectin: ✗
- Oxalate: ✗
- Salicylates: ✗

DASH Diet (Hypertension): A few sources point to goji berries lowering blood pressure; however, be aware that these berries may react to certain medications such as blood thinners, diabetes and blood pressure medication (source: *Healthline*). They're also higher in sodium and sugar than other berries, so eat in moderation. *Saturated fat content: 0.4g (per 100g), Sodium content: 298mg (per 100g), 13% daily value based on a 2,000 calorie diet, Sugar content: 46g (per 100g)* (source: *Nutrition Value*).

Diverticulitis: No solid foods can be eaten at stage one, the clear liquids diet. Allowed on the high-fiber diet.

Histamine: Allowed.

Lectins: A part of the nightshade family which are high in lectins.

Oxalates: High.

Salicylates: While there isn't any information available specifically related to the amount of salicylates in goji berries, berries in general contain a high content. This leads us to conclude that this superfood for some, is not a superfood for salicylate sufferers. So - it is best avoided or consumed in small amounts.

Goose (organic, freshly cooked)

- DASH: Fat: ✗ Sodium: ✓ Sugar: ✓
- Diverticulitis: Stage 1: ✗ Stage 2: ✓ Stage 3: ✗
- Histamine: ✓
- Lectin: ✓
- Oxalate: ✓
- Salicylates: ✓

DASH Diet (Hypertension): One source notes the high nutrition content in goose meat but doesn't recommend it for people with high blood pressure. The legs and skin of geese have the highest fat content so remove these before eating. Go for the breast meat as this has less fat (source: *Health and Social Services, Government of Northwest Territories*). *Saturated fat content: 4.56g (per 100g), Sodium content: 76mg (per 100g), 3% daily value based on a 2,000 calorie diet, Sugar content: N/A (per 100g)* (source: *Fatsecret Platform API*).

Diverticulitis: No solid foods can be eaten at stage one, the clear liquids diet. Poultry contains no fiber, so goose is allowed on a low-fiber diet.

Histamine: Tolerated.

Lectins: Accepted. Opt for pasture-raised geese.

Oxalates: See "Meat"

Salicylates: See "Meat"

Gooseberry, gooseberries

- DASH: Fat: ✓ Sodium: ✓ Sugar: ✓
- Diverticulitis: Stage 1: ✗ Stage 2: ✗ Stage 3: ✓
- Histamine: ✓
- Lectin: 🤔
- Oxalate: ✗
- Salicylates: ✗

DASH Diet (Hypertension): A soft fruit allowed on the DASH diet. According to Eat Delights' blog, gooseberries taste similar to strawberries, apples and grapes. What an interesting combination. *Saturated fat content: 0.038g (per 100g), Sodium content: 1mg (per 100g), less than 1% daily value based on a 2,000 calorie diet, Sugar content: N/A (per 100g).*

Diverticulitis: No solid foods can be eaten at stage one, the clear liquids diet. Allowed on the high-fiber diet.

Histamine: Tolerated.

Lectins: Not a lot of information out there, but since gooseberries are related to currants, we think they could also be a source of lectins. Test carefully.

Oxalates: Indian gooseberries are high in oxalate.

Salicylates: Gooseberries are thought to be high in salicylates.

Gouda cheese

- DASH: Fat: ✗ Sodium: ✗ Sugar: ✓
- Diverticulitis: Stage 1: ✗ Stage 2: ✓ Stage 3: ✗
- Histamine: ✗
- Lectin: ✗
- Oxalate: ✓
- Salicylates: ✓

DASH Diet (Hypertension): Low in sugar but thought to be high in saturated fat and sodium content. Avoid. Livestrong's website suggests going for Swiss, Feta or Parmesan if you want to eat cheese. *Saturated fat content: 18g (per 100g), Sodium content: 819 mg (per 100g) 34% daily value based on a 2,000 calorie diet, Sugar content: 2.2g (per 100g).*

Diverticulitis: No solid foods can be eaten at stage one, the clear liquids diet. Cheese contains no fiber, so they're allowed on the low-fiber diet.

Histamine: See general comments under 'Cheese'.

Lectins: Avoid. It's thought that Gouda cheese is made from casein proteins which are high in lectins.

Oxalates: See cheese.

Salicylates: Most cheeses are thought to be very low in salicylates. Choose cheeses made from 100 percent grass-fed animals for the highest level of nutrients and avoid processed types that may contain salicylates and other potentially harmful ingredients.

Grapefruit

- DASH: Fat: ✓ Sodium: ✓ Sugar: ✗
- Diverticulitis: Stage 1: ✗ Stage 2: ✗ Stage 3: ✓
- Histamine: ✗
- Lectin: 😕
- Oxalate: ✗
- Salicylates: ✗

DASH Diet (Hypertension): Low in saturated fat and sodium content but high in sugar. Eat in moderation. Watch out if you're taking medication, as grapefruit may interfere with blood pressure medication (source: *Havard Health*). *Saturated fat content: 0g (per 100g), Sodium content: 0mg (per 100g), Sugar content: 7g (per 100g).*

Diverticulitis: No solid foods can be eaten at stage one, the clear liquids diet. Allowed on the high-fiber diet.

Histamine: While many foods are on the allowed list with histamine intolerance, this one is a disappointment - grapefruit normally seems to cause a reaction.

Lectins: Moderate lectin content, but given the high antioxidants and enormous health benefits, these can be enjoyed in moderation.

Oxalates: Very high. Thought to be one of the highest oxalate fruits, unfortunately.

Salicylates: Analysis from the Food Research Institute found no detectable salicylates in grapefruit; however, several reliable sources, including Millhouse Medical Center and WebMD, consider it to have a high amount. Eat in moderation until you know how it will affect you.

Grapes

- DASH: Fat: ✓ Sodium: ✓ Sugar: ✗
- Diverticulitis: Stage 1: ✗ Stage 2: ✓ Stage 3: ✗
- Histamine: 😕
- Lectin: 😕
- Oxalate: ✓
- Salicylates: ✗

DASH Diet (Hypertension): Low in saturated fat and sodium content but high in sugar. Limit grapes in your meal plan. *Saturated fat content: 0.1g (per 100g), Sodium content: 2mg (per 100g), less than 1% daily value based on a 2,000 calorie diet, Sugar content: 16g (per 100g).*

Diverticulitis: No solid foods can be eaten at stage one, the clear liquids diet. Grapes contain very little fiber, so they're allowed on the low-fiber diet.

Histamine: Some lists don't agree that grapes are low in histamine. In addition, they are very high in sugar.

Lectins: Moderate lectin content. Limit grapes because of their high sugar levels. Note that the nutrition content of grapes depends on how they're grown. For example, it's thought that grapes grown at a higher altitude have more exposure to the sun so they contain higher levels of Polyphenols (anti-oxidants) (source: *Katherine Senko: Polyphenols in Wine*).

Oxalates: Thought to be low in oxalate. However, they are very high in sugar.

Salicylates: Grapes vary in their salicylate content depending on the type, which may be why we've found conflicting information among reliable sites. Some of our favorite sources categorize grapes in general as "high", with numerous others rating red grapes in particular with a much higher content than green, ranging between .49 mg and 1 mg per 100 g. Our best advice based on information is to choose green grapes and consume just a small amount until you know how they will affect you.

Green beans

- DASH: Fat: ✓ Sodium: ✓ Sugar: ✓
- Diverticulitis: Stage 1: ✗ Stage 2: ✗ Stage 3: ✓
- Histamine: ✗
- Lectin: ✗
- Oxalate: ✓
- Salicylates: 😕

DASH Diet (Hypertension): Allowed. Try roasting green beans with herbs, garlic and olive oil — it tastes delicious. Eat 4-5 servings of vegetables a day. *Saturated fat content: 0g (per 100g), Sodium content: 6mg (per 100g), less than 1% daily value based on a 2,000 calorie diet, Sugar content: N/A (per 100g).*

Diverticulitis: No solid foods can be eaten at stage one, the clear liquids diet. Allowed on the high-fiber diet.

Histamine: See "beans"

Lectins: High in lectins. One to put on your 'avoid' list. If you want to eat beans, the FDA recommends boiling them for 30 minutes to reduce the lectin content. Avoid canned beans as most of these haven't been soaked or cooked to reduce lectin content.

Oxalates: See "beans"

Salicylates: See "beans"

Green peas

- DASH: Fat: ✓ Sodium: ✓ Sugar: ✗
- Diverticulitis: Stage 1: ✗ Stage 2: ✗ Stage 3: ✓
- Histamine: 😕
- Lectin: 😕
- Oxalate: ✓
- Salicylates: ✓

DASH Diet (Hypertension): Low in saturated fat and sodium content but high in sugar. Multiple sources allow green peas on the DASH diet. *Saturated fat content: 0.1g (per 100g), Sodium content: 5mg (per 100g), less than 1% daily value based on a 2,000 calorie diet, Sugar content: 6g (per 100g).*

Diverticulitis: No solid foods can be eaten at stage one, the clear liquids diet. Allowed on the high-fiber diet.

Histamine: Peas are a weird one. We seem to tolerate them well, however having canvassed the histamine community, many people do struggle with them. Mast Cell 360 lists green split peas and yellow split peas as low histamine, just "peas" as high histamine.

Lectins: Mixed opinion. Some say they contain low levels of lectins and are safe to eat. However, others believe they may interfere with gut absorption. A study found that soaking peas *"significantly decreased the contents of lectins"* (source: *Shi L, Arntfield SD, Nickerson M. Changes in levels of phytic acid, lectins and oxalates during soaking and cooking of Canadian pulses*). Limit consumption and test carefully initially.

Oxalates: Peas are considered low in oxalate, with only 1 mg of oxalate per half cup (source: *St. Joseph's Healthcare Hamilton*).

Salicylates: Dried peas contain only trace amounts of salicylates, while fresh green peas may have a low amount of up to .25 mg per 100 g. Note that the emoji is based on dried peas or fresh green peas only as snow peas may contain a higher level. As well as being thought to be low in salicylates, green peas are an excellent source of vitamin C as well as containing a good amount of protein, magnesium, iron, and fiber.

Green tea

- DASH: Fat: ✓ Sodium: ✓ Sugar: ✓
- Diverticulitis: Stage 1: ✓ Stage 2: ✓ Stage 3: ✗
- Histamine: 😕
- Lectin: ✓
- Oxalate: 😕
- Salicylates: ✗

DASH Diet (Hypertension): Allowed. The flavonoids in green tea have been shown to lower LDL cholesterol levels (source: *Dietician UK*). *Saturated fat content: 0.002g (per 100g), Sodium content: 1mg (per 100g), less than 1% daily value based on a 2,000 calorie diet, Sugar content: 0g (per 100g).*

Diverticulitis: Tea with no milk or cream is allowed at stage one, the clear liquid diet. Also allowed on the low-fiber diet.

Histamine: Test carefully.

Lectins: It's thought that tea is tolerated on a low-lectin diet. A study found that green tea *"can be beneficial for people exposed to plant lectins"* as it *"alleviates hepatic inflammatory damage and immunological reaction"* in mice. The green tea polyphenols (antioxidants) *"exert protective effects"* (source: *Wang D, Zhang M, Wang T, Liu T, Guo Y, Granato D. Green tea polyphenols mitigate the plant lectins-induced liver inflammation and immunological reaction in C57BL/6 mice via NLRP3 and Nrf2 signaling pathways*).

Oxalates: Wildly varies depending on the tea and the investigative source.

Research shows that the amount of oxalate measured for black tea varies from 2.7 to 4.8 mg/240 mL (one cup) of tea infused for 1–5 min, whereas the amount of oxalate in green tea ranges from 2.08 to 34.94 mg/250 mL of tea (source: *US National Library of Medicine*). However, the amount of oxalate in green tea depends on its origin, quality, preparation, and harvest time, thus probably explaining why some studies report a higher oxalate concentration in black tea than in green tea.

Salicylates: Most teas, including green tea, according to WebMD, contain a very high level of salicylates.

Guava

- DASH: Fat: ✓ Sodium: ✓ Sugar: ✗
- Diverticulitis: Stage 1: ✗ Stage 2: ✗ Stage 3: ✓
- Histamine: ✗
- Lectin: 🤔
- Oxalate: ✗
- Salicylates: ✗

DASH Diet (Hypertension): Low in saturated fat and sodium content but high in sugar. Guava is high in potassium, and one study found *"120 people who ate guava before each meal for 12 weeks saw a reduction in total cholesterol and blood pressure, and experienced an increase in good (HDL) cholesterol."* (source: *Singh RB, Rastogi SS, Singh R, Ghosh S, Niaz MA. Effects of guava intake on serum total and high-density lipoprotein cholesterol levels and on systemic blood pressure. Am J Cardiol.*) *Saturated fat content: 0.3g (per 100g), Sodium content: 2mg (per 100g), less than 1% daily value based on a 2,000 calorie diet, Sugar content: 9g (per 100g).*

Diverticulitis: No solid foods can be eaten at stage one, the clear liquids diet. Guava is a good source of fiber. Allowed on the high-fiber diet.

Histamine: Avoid.

Lectins: Thought to contain moderate lectins.

Oxalates: High. Thought to change in oxalate content depending on ripeness.

Salicylates: Whether fresh or canned, guava is very high in salicylates.

Ham (dried, cured)

- DASH: Fat: ✗ Sodium: ✗ Sugar: ✓
- Diverticulitis: Stage 1: ✗ Stage 2: ✓ Stage 3: ✗
- Histamine: ✗
- Lectin: ✓
- Oxalate: ✓
- Salicylates: ✗

DASH Diet (Hypertension): Low in sugar but thought to be high in saturated fat and sodium content. Ham is processed red meat. The American Institute of Cancer Research reported a link between cancer and processed meat. Avoid on the DASH diet. *Saturated fat content: 1.8g (per 100g), Sodium content: 1,203mg (per 100g) 50% daily value based on a 2,000 calorie diet, Sugar content: 0g (per 100g).*

Diverticulitis: No solid foods can be eaten at stage one, the clear liquids diet. Meat contains no fiber, so ham is allowed on the low-fiber diet.

Histamine: Avoid processed meat, dried meat and cured meat. It will make your histamine intolerance worse.

Lectins: Tolerated. Ensure these are grass-fed.

Oxalates: Low oxalate. However, eating large portions of meat can potentially increase the risk of kidney stones.

Salicylates: While most meats do not contain salicylates, cured meats typically contain additives that make them best avoided. See "Dry-Cured Meats"

Hazelnut

- DASH: Fat: ✗ Sodium: ✓ Sugar: ✓
- Diverticulitis: Stage 1: ✗ Stage 2: ✗ Stage 3: ✓
- Histamine: 😖
- Lectin: ✓
- Oxalate: ✗
- Salicylates: 😖

DASH Diet (Hypertension): Ensure you eat no more than 4-5 servings a week and go for unsalted nuts. Eating Well's website notes hazelnuts as part of the DASH diet and a heart-healthy lifestyle. *Saturated fat content: 4.5g (per 100g), Sodium content: 0mg (per 100g), Sugar content: 4.3g (per 100g).*

Diverticulitis: No solid foods can be eaten at stage one, the clear liquids diet. Allowed on the high-fiber diet.

Histamine: Test carefully, but we consider it one of the best nuts.

Lectins: Tolerated. A great alternative to peanuts.

Oxalates: High, best avoided. Nuts are high in oxalates.

Salicylates: According to multiple resources, hazelnuts have a low amount of salicylates. Hazelnuts are an outstanding source of vitamin E and magnesium, and they are high in calories. As we cannot be 100 percent sure based on information as to the exact amount of salicylates in hazelnuts, eat in limited amounts or test carefully.

Hemp seeds (Cannabis sativa)

- DASH: Fat: ✗ Sodium: ✓ Sugar: ✓
- Diverticulitis: Stage 1: ✗ Stage 2: ✗ Stage 3: ✓
- Histamine: ✓
- Lectin: ✓
- Oxalate: ✓
- Salicylates: 😖

DASH Diet (Hypertension): They're full of omega-3 fatty acids, which we need for a healthy heart. Ensure you eat no more than 4-5 servings a week. *Saturated fat content: 4.6g (per 100g), Sodium content: 5mg (per 100g), less than 1% daily value based on a 2,000 calorie diet, Sugar content: 1.5g (per 100g)* (source: *Nutrition Value*).

Diverticulitis: No solid foods can be eaten at stage one, the clear liquids diet. Allowed on the high-fiber diet.

Histamine: We love hemp derivatives and CBD products too.

Lectins: Seeds usually contain lectins but not hemp seeds. These are thought to be very low or free of lectins.

Oxalates: Nuts and seeds are high in oxalates, but hemp seeds are thought to be a better choice. They contain just 3 mg oxalate per 2 tablespoons (source: *https://www.thekidneydietitian.org/low-oxalate-nuts/*).

Salicylates: Most seeds contain a low-to-moderate amount of salicylates. We have scoured the Internet for information related to hemp seeds and could not find specific details. Our research yielded some information on hemp seed oil, which contained trace amounts of salicylates, reported in a lab analysis titled The Composition of Hemp Seed Oil and Its Potential as an Important Source of Nutrition.

Herbal tea

- DASH: Fat: ✓ Sodium: ✓ Sugar: ✗
- Diverticulitis: Stage 1: ✓ Stage 2: ✓ Stage 3: ✗
- Histamine: 😐
- Lectin: ✓
- Oxalate: 😐
- Salicylates: ✗

DASH Diet (Hypertension): Low in saturated fat and sodium content but high in sugar. Check the nutrition labels and make sure the herbal tea is unsweetened. Drink in moderation. *Saturated fat content: 0.3g (per 100g), Sodium content: 3mg (per 100g) less than 1% daily value based on a 2,000 calorie diet, Sugar content: 6g (per 100g).*

Diverticulitis: Tea with no milk or cream is allowed at stage one, the clear liquid diet. Also allowed on the low-fiber diet.

Histamine: Depends on the tea and the individual ingredients. Please look up the individual ingredients in our list.

Lectins: It's thought that tea is acceptable on a low-lectin diet.

Oxalates: Depends on the tea and the individual ingredients. Please look up the individual ingredients on our list. Some teas, including black teas, are thought to accumulate many oxalates, resulting in a recommendation to eliminate black tea from your diet if you form oxalate stones (source: *nature.com*). In a 2003 study, researchers from New Zealand discovered a 'tea hack'. They noted; *"These studies show that consuming black tea on a daily basis will lead to a moderate intake of soluble oxalate each day, however the consumption of tea with milk on a regular basis will result in the absorption of very little oxalate from tea."*

Salicylates: Many, if not most herbal teas are thought to contain a very high level of salicylates. See individual ingredients and teas for more details.

Honey

- DASH: Fat: ✓ Sodium: ✓ Sugar: ✗
- Diverticulitis: Stage 1: ✓ Stage 2: ✓ Stage 3: ✗
- Histamine: ✓
- Lectin: ✓
- Oxalate: ✓
- Salicylates: ✗

DASH Diet (Hypertension): Low in saturated fat and sodium content but high in sugar. Avoid adding sugar to your diet, even if it's honey. Eat in moderation. *Saturated fat content: 0g (per 100g), Sodium content: 4mg (per 100g), less than 1% daily value based on a 2,000 calorie diet, Sugar content: 82g (per 100g).*

Diverticulitis: Contains very little fiber. Allowed on the low-fiber diet.

Histamine: Tolerated.

Lectins: Acceptable however, note the high sugar content. Eat in moderation.

Oxalates: See sweeteners.

Salicylates: High in salicylates with the exact level depending on the brand. Different kinds of honey are thought to range between 2.5mg and over 10 mg of salicylates per 100 g, all considered high.

Horseradish

- DASH: Fat: ✓ Sodium: ✗ Sugar: ✗
- Diverticulitis: Stage 1: ✗ Stage 2: ✗ Stage 3: ✓
- Histamine: 😣
- Lectin: ✓
- Oxalate: ✓
- Salicylates: ✓

DASH Diet (Hypertension): Whilst this root veg is thought to help reduce inflammation, fight cell damage and improve respiratory health (source: *WebMD*), it's relatively high in sodium and sugar. Limit consumption. *Saturated fat content: 0.09g (per 100g), Sodium content: 314 mg (per 100g), 14% daily value based on a 2,000 calorie diet, Sugar content: 7.99g (per 100g)* (source: *Fatsecret Platform API*).

Diverticulitis: No solid foods can be eaten at stage one, the clear liquids diet. Allowed on the high-fiber diet.

Histamine: Test carefully.

Lectins: Falls under the cruciferous vegetable family (includes broccoli, kale, cabbage, radish etc.). These are considered low-lectin and rich in vitamin C, folate and fiber.

Oxalates: Low oxalate. Sally K. Norton recommends it as a substitute for high-oxalate herbs and spices: *"Try prepared horseradish more often. It is great with beef and seafood."*

Salicylates: Horseradish contains a low amount of salicylates, ranging from .15 to .25 mg per 100g.

Juniper berries

- DASH: Fat: ✓ Sodium: ✓ Sugar: ✓
- Diverticulitis: Stage 1: ✗ Stage 2: ✗ Stage 3: ✓
- Histamine: ✓
- Lectin: 😣
- Oxalate: ✓
- Salicylates: No information

Don't be confused by its name, despite looking like blueberries, these aren't consumed like berries because of the bitterness.

DASH Diet (Hypertension): Allowed. They're packed full of antioxidants too. *Saturated fat content: 0g (per 100g), Sodium content: N/A (per 100g), Sugar content: 4.2g (per 100g)* (source: *Nutrition Value*).

Diverticulitis: No solid foods can be eaten at stage one, the clear liquids diet. Allowed on the high-fiber diet.

Histamine: Acceptable.

Lectins: Used as a bitter spice for a range of dishes, we know that spices may be consumed on a low-lectin diet, so perhaps these may also be tolerated.

Oxalates: Juniper berries are considered lithotriptic, which means that they help to dissolve and discharge urinary stones once they have formed. (source: *Journal of the Mazandaran University of Medical Sciences*).

Salicylates: There is no information on the content of salicylates.

Kale

- DASH: Fat: ✓ Sodium: ✓ Sugar: ✓
- Diverticulitis: Stage 1: ✗ Stage 2: ✗ Stage 3: ✓
- Histamine: ✓
- Lectin: ✓
- Oxalate: ✓
- Salicylates: 😷

DASH Diet (Hypertension): Allowed. Kale is thought to help lower blood pressure naturally. Have you tried kale chips? They're a great crispy snack and a healthy alternative to potato chips. Consume 4-5 servings of vegetables a day. *Saturated fat content: 0.091g (per 100g), Sodium content: 43mg (per 100g), 2% daily value based on a 2,000 calorie diet, Sugar content: N/A (per 100g)* (source: *Fatsecret Platform API*).

Diverticulitis: No solid foods can be eaten at stage one, the clear liquids diet. Allowed on the high-fiber diet.

Histamine: Kale is listed as lower histamine on the major sites.

Lectins: Falls under the cruciferous vegetable family (includes broccoli, Brussel sprouts, cabbage, radish etc.). These are thought to be low-lectin and rich in vitamin C, folate and fiber.

Oxalates: Kale is thought to be low in oxalate, which makes it a good veggie choice.

Salicylates: Kale is one reason we wrote this book. Opinion differs significantly on kale and salicylates and that makes it a frustrating ingredient for sufferers of salicylate intolerance. Guaranteeing the amount of salicylates in kale is impossible. This popular superfood is ranked anywhere from low to high depending on which online source you consult, and for us, kale is always followed by a question mark. As it is like chard, also known as *Roman kale* which is likely to contain a high level, we recommend avoiding or starting with a very limited amount until you know how your body will react.

Kefir

- DASH: Fat: ✗ Sodium: ✓ Sugar: ✓
- Diverticulitis: Stage 1: ✗ Stage 2: ✓ Stage 3: ✗
- Histamine: ✗
- Lectin: ✗
- Oxalate: ✓
- Salicylates: ✓
- Kefir is a fermented milk product.

DASH Diet (Hypertension): Very high in fat — best to avoid however, a source suggests drinking kefir may have a positive effect on blood pressure. A study has shown traditional kefir may help control blood cholesterol levels however, more studies need to be carried out as traditional kefir may differ from commercial kefir (source: *https://clinicaltrials.gov/ct2/show/NCT04247139*).

Diverticulitis: Avoid at stage one, the clear liquid diet as kefir is made of milk causes flare-ups. All liquids should be clear. It contains no fiber, so allowed on a low-fiber diet.

Histamine: High histamine as fermented. This could be lower histamine if you make it yourself with histamine-friendly bacteria.

Lectins: Avoid. Contains A1 casein protein.

Oxalates: Very low in oxalates. Cow's milk doesn't have oxalate, so if kefir is made from cow's milk, it's a good choice. Note, that kefir can also be made from other sources.

Salicylates: As cow's milk, goat's milk, and other milk from animals are free of salicylates, provided it is made from one of these sources, we believe kefir should be as well. It's also loaded with probiotics that are good for your gut.

Kelp

- DASH: Fat: ✓ Sodium: ✗ Sugar: ✓
- Diverticulitis: Stage 1: ✗ Stage 2: ✗ Stage 3: ✓
- Histamine: ✗
- Lectin: ✓
- Oxalate: 🤢
- Salicylates: ✗

DASH Diet (Hypertension): Winchester Hospital notes kelp has been used to "*promote weight loss and lower blood pressure*", but there isn't enough study to show the benefits of kelp in treating health problems. Watch the sodium content. *Saturated fat content: 0.2g (per 100g), Sodium content: 233 mg (per 100g), 10% daily value based on a 2,000 calorie diet, Sugar content: 0.6g (per 100g)* (source: *Nutrition Value*).

Diverticulitis: No solid foods can be eaten at stage one, the clear liquids diet. Allowed on the high-fiber diet.

Histamine: Avoid.

Lectins: Thought to be low-lectin.

Oxalates: Sometimes recommended as a nutrient to prevent kidney stones. This is because it's very high in calcium. Kelp is a type of seaweed, but oxalate content can vary from very high to very low depending on the specific seaweed.

Salicylates: Kelp is a type of brown seaweed, and as seaweed is high in salicylates, it should be avoided or consumed in minimal amounts.

Kiwi

- DASH: Fat: ✓ Sodium: ✓ Sugar: ✗
- Diverticulitis: Stage 1: ✗ Stage 2: ✗ Stage 3: ✓
- Histamine: ✗
- Lectin: ✓
- Oxalate: ✗
- Salicylates: ✗

DASH Diet (Hypertension): Low in saturated fat and sodium content but high in sugar. Kiwis are thought to be rich in vitamin C, which may improve blood pressure. A study on men and women with moderately elevated blood pressure found: "*Intake of three kiwifruits was associated with lower systolic and diastolic 24-h BP compared with one apple a day.*" (source: *Svendsen M, Tonstad S, Heggen E, Pedersen TR, Seljeflot I, Bøhn SK, Bastani NE, Blomhoff R, Holme IM, Klemsdal TO. The effect of kiwifruit consumption on blood pressure in subjects with moderately elevated blood pressure: a randomized, controlled study. Blood Press. 2015*). *Saturated fat content: 0g (per 100g), Sodium content: 3mg (per 100g), less than 1% daily value based on a 2,000 calorie diet, Sugar content: 9g (per 100g).*

Diverticulitis: No solid foods can be eaten at stage one, the clear liquids diet. Allowed on the high-fiber diet

Histamine: High histamine, however, others disagree so approach cautiously.

Lectins: Health Canal's website refers to kiwi as a *"natural lectin blocker"* because kiwi increases mucin production in our bodies. Mucin contains sialic acid, which blocks lectins from causing harm to our digestive system. Best to eat when kiwi is in season.

Oxalates: Very high.

Salicylates: Kiwi contains a moderate to a high amount of salicylates depending on the analysis, making it best to avoid caution.

Kohlrabi

- DASH: Fat: ✓ Sodium: ✓ Sugar: ✓
- Diverticulitis: Stage 1: ✗ Stage 2: ✗ Stage 3: ✓
- Histamine: 😐
- Lectin: ✓
- Oxalate: ✓
- Salicylates: ✓

A type of cultivar of wild cabbage in the same species as cabbage and Brussels sprouts. Also known as *German turnip*. Like cabbage, Cook For Your Life's blog notes kohlrabi may be eaten raw, steamed or blanched.

DASH Diet (Hypertension): Allowed. *Saturated fat content: 0g (per 100g), Sodium content: 20mg (per 100g) less than 1% daily value based on a 2,000 calorie diet, Sugar content: 2.6g (per 100g).*

Diverticulitis: No solid foods can be eaten at stage one, the clear liquids diet. Allowed on the high-fiber diet.

Histamine: Test carefully.

Lectins: Thought to be low-lectin.

Oxalates: Thought to be low in oxalate.

Salicylates: While there isn't much information available on it in relation to salicylates, a few reliable sources rank it low in salicylates. Because of kohlrabi's relation to the other low salicylate vegetables, it is likely safe for sensitive individuals, however, eat in small amounts until you know how it will affect you.

Lamb

- DASH: Fat: 😐 Sodium: ✓ Sugar: ✓
- Diverticulitis: Stage 1: ✗ Stage 2: ✓ Stage 3: ✗
- Histamine: ✓
- Lectin: ✓
- Oxalate: ✓
- Salicylates: ✓

DASH Diet (Hypertension): High in fat. Limit consumption of red meat such as lamb. *Saturated fat content: 9g (per 100g), 45% daily value based on a 2,000 calorie diet, Sodium content: 72mg (per 100g) 3% daily value based on a 2,000 calorie diet, Sugar content: 0g (per 100g).*

Diverticulitis: No solid foods can be eaten at stage one, the clear liquids diet. Meat contains no fiber so lamb is allowed on the low-fiber diet.

Histamine: Must be organic and fresh. No leftovers.

Lectins: Tolerated. Opt for grass-fed lamb.

Oxalates: Low oxalate. See comments about meat.

Salicylates: See "Meat"

Lamb's lettuce, corn salad
- DASH: Fat: ✔ Sodium: ✘ Sugar: ✔
- Diverticulitis: Stage 1: ✘ Stage 2: ✘ Stage 3: ✔
- Histamine: ✔
- Lectin: ✘
- Oxalate: ✔
- Salicylates: 💀

Corn salad is usually made with corn kernels, tomatoes, cucumbers, feta and herbs.

DASH Diet (Hypertension): Thought to be allowed on the DASH diet as it's high in potassium which protects against cardiovascular disease. It's great for warm weather too. Why not take this healthy dish with you on your next picnic? *Saturated fat content: 1g (per 100g), Sodium content: 177.5mg (per 100g), 7% daily value based on a 2,000 calorie diet, Sugar content: 4g (per 100g)* (source: Nutritionix).

Diverticulitis: No solid foods can be eaten at stage one, the clear liquids diet. Allowed on the high-fiber diet.

Histamine: Tolerated.

Lectins: Corn Salad is made with corn kernels, and all corn foods should be avoided.

Oxalates: Low oxalate.

Salicylates: See "Lettuce"

Lard
- DASH: Fat: ✘ Sodium: ✔ Sugar: ✔
- Diverticulitis: Stage 1: ✘ Stage 2: ✔ Stage 3: ✘
- Histamine: ✔
- Lectin: ✔
- Oxalate: ✔
- Salicylates: ✔

DASH Diet (Hypertension): Lard is a source of fat — watch your intake as too much fat will raise your blood pressure. Interesting fact: lard has 20% less saturated fat than butter (source: *Supermarket Guru*). Other sources suggest cooking with lard instead of butter. *Saturated fat content: 32g (per 100g), Sodium content: 27mg (per 100g), 1% daily value based on a 2,000 calorie diet, Sugar content: 0g (per 100g).*

Diverticulitis: No solid foods can be eaten at stage one, the clear liquids diet. It contains no fiber, so allowed on a low-fiber diet.

Histamine: Fresh or frozen only.

Lectins: A low-lectin fat made of 100% pork fat from the kidneys and back.

Oxalates: Very low, less than 5 mg per 100 grams (source: *University of Virginia*).

Salicylates: Lard is thought to be low in salicylates. It has about half as much saturated fat as butter but double the amount found in olive oil. A good choice for cooking.

Leek

- DASH: Fat: ✓ Sodium: ✓ Sugar: ✓
- Diverticulitis: Stage 1: ✗ Stage 2: ✗ Stage 3: ✓
- Histamine: 😖
- Lectin: ✓
- Oxalate: 😖
- Salicylates: ✓

DASH Diet (Hypertension): Low in calories and allowed on the DASH diet. Eat 4-5 servings of vegetables a day. *Saturated fat content: 0g (per 100g), Sodium content: 20mg (per 100g), less than 1% daily value based on a 2,000 calorie diet, Sugar content: 3.9g (per 100g).*

Diverticulitis: No solid foods can be eaten at stage one, the clear liquids diet. Allowed on the high-fiber diet.

Histamine: Likely to be low histamine. Test carefully.

Lectins: Contains little lectin.

Oxalates: Leeks contain 89.0 mg of oxalate per 100 grams (source: *UPMC*). Consume moderately or avoid it if you're on a low-oxalate diet.

Salicylates: Leeks are considered generally low in salicylates.

Lemon

- DASH: Fat: ✓ Sodium: ✓ Sugar: ✓
- Diverticulitis: Stage 1: ✓ Stage 2: ✗ Stage 3: ✓
- Histamine: ✗
- Lectin: 😖
- Oxalate: 😖
- Salicylates: 😖

DASH Diet (Hypertension): Allowed. Lemon juice is great for adding flavor to your dish. *Saturated fat content: 0g (per 100g), Sodium content: 2mg (per 100g) less than 1% daily value based on a 2,000 calorie diet, Sugar content: 2.5g (per 100g).*

Diverticulitis: Lemon juice is allowed if it's clear with no seeds and pulp. Lemon is a rich source of fiber so allowed on a high-fiber diet.

Histamine: see "citrus fruit"

Lectins: These are a source of lectins, but given the high antioxidants, the benefits outweigh the negatives. It's thought that these can be enjoyed in moderation. Test carefully.

Oxalates: A confusing one. Lemon is often considered to be low oxalate. However, lemon peels are quite high in oxalate - 83.0 mg per 100 grams - and lemon juice has just 1.0 mg per 100 g (source: *UPMC*).

Salicylates: Most of our research has shown that lemons are low in salicylates, with up to .25 mg per 100 g. However, some sources categorize this sour fruit as "moderate,". Please note that there is anecdotal evidence from several sensitive individuals in the salicylate world reporting no negative effects from lemon or lemon juice. This conflicting information makes it difficult to accurately rate lemons, hence test carefully.

Lentils

- DASH: Fat: ✓ Sodium: ✓ Sugar: ✓

- Diverticulitis: Stage 1: ✗ Stage 2: ✗ Stage 3: ✓
- Histamine: ✗
- Lectin: ✗
- Oxalate: ✓
- Salicylates: ✓

DASH Diet (Hypertension): Allowed. A daily cup of lentils is thought to *"keep your blood pressure in check"* (source: WebMD). *Saturated fat content: 0.1g (per 100g), Sodium content: 2mg (per 100g), less than 1% daily value based on a 2,000 calorie diet, Sugar content: 1.8g (per 100g).*

Diverticulitis: No solid foods can be eaten at stage one, the clear liquids diet. Allowed on the high-fiber diet.

Histamine: Some say lentils are actually low histamine, although high if tinned. We find them to be high histamine

Lectins: High in lectins. Lentils are thought to be especially high in lectins.

Oxalates: Boiled lentils have low-to-moderate oxalate content.

Salicylates: Free or very low in salicylates, lentils are a reliable source of plant-based protein on a low-salicylate diet.

Lettuce

- DASH: Fat: ✓ Sodium: ✓ Sugar: ✓
- Diverticulitis: Stage 1: ✗ Stage 2: ✓ Stage 3: ✗
- Histamine: ✓
- Lectin: ✓
- Oxalate: ✓
- Salicylates: ✓

DASH Diet (Hypertension): Allowed. Eat 4-5 servings of vegetables a day. *Saturated fat content: 0g (per 100g), Sodium content: 28mg (per 100g), 1% daily value based on a 2,000 calorie diet, Sugar content: 0.8g (per 100g).*

Diverticulitis: No solid foods can be eaten at stage one, the clear liquids diet. Lettuce is low in fiber so allowed on a low-fiber diet.

Histamine: Tolerated.

Lectins: Thought to be low-lectin.

Oxalates: All kinds of lettuce are thought to be low in oxalates.

Salicylates: The short answer is - it depends on the lettuce. Iceberg is the most common type of lettuce, and it's thought to contain only a negligible amount of salicylates. Other lettuces can have higher levels of salicylates, such as lamb's lettuce and butterhead lettuce, which have a moderate level ranging from .25 to .49 mg per 100 g.

Lime

- DASH: Fat: ✓ Sodium: ✓ Sugar: ✓
- Diverticulitis: Stage 1: ✓ Stage 2: ✗ Stage 3: ✓
- Histamine: ✗
- Lectin: 🤔
- Oxalate: 🤔
- Salicylates: ✓

DASH Diet (Hypertension): Allowed. Citrus fruits contain vitamins and minerals and may lower your blood pressure. *Saturated fat content: 0g (per 100g), Sodium content: 2mg (per 100g), less than 1% daily value based on a 2,000 calorie diet, Sugar content: 1.7g (per 100g).*

Diverticulitis: Lime juice is allowed if it's clear with no seeds and pulp. Allowed on the high-fiber diet.

Histamine: Avoid. More notes under 'Citrus'.

Lectins: These are a source of lectins, but given the high antioxidants, the benefits outweigh the negatives. It's thought that these can be enjoyed in moderation. Test carefully.

Oxalates: Lime juice is thought to contain low amounts of oxalates (between 2-5mg of oxalates per 100 grams, according to various sources). It should be noted there is some divergence between lists. Lime peels contain 110 mg per gram (source: *UPMC*). It's not often a person eats a lot of lime peel, but this would be something to be avoided.

Salicylates: Both limes and lime juice contain very low levels of salicylates, according to multiple reliable sources.

Liquor

- DASH: Fat: ✓ Sodium: ✓ Sugar: ✓
- Diverticulitis: Stage 1: ✗ Stage 2: ✗ Stage 3: ✗
- Histamine: ✗
- Lectin: 😕
- Oxalate: ✓
- Salicylates: ✗

DASH Diet (Hypertension): Avoid sweetened liquor. Liquor is allowed on the DASH diet, but many sources advise drinking alcohol sparingly. *Saturated fat content: 0g (per 100g), Sodium content: 1mg (per 100g), less than 1% daily value based on a 2,000 calorie diet, Sugar content: 0g (per 100g).*

Diverticulitis: See alcohol.

Histamine: See alcohol.

Lectins: Aged liquors are acceptable on a low-lectin diet.

Oxalates: See alcohol.

Salicylates: Alcoholic beverages contain a high level of salicylates.

Liquorice

- DASH: Fat: ✗ Sodium: ✗ Sugar: ✗
- Diverticulitis: Stage 1: ✗ Stage 2: ✓ Stage 3: ✗
- Histamine: ✗
- Lectin: 😕
- Oxalate: ✗
- Salicylates: ✗

Also known as *licorice*. Avoid large quantities of liquorice as this could increase blood pressure and arrhythmia (source: *NHS*).

DASH Diet (Hypertension): Avoid. The NHS notes: *"Eating more than 57g (2 ounces) of black liquorice a day for at least 2 weeks could lead to potentially serious health problems, such as an increase in blood pressure and an irregular* heart rhythm (arrhythmia)." Saturated fat content: 1.3g (per 100g), Sodium content: 162mg (per 100g), 7% daily value based on a 2,000 calorie diet, Sugar content: 40g (per 100g).

Diverticulitis: No solid foods can be eaten at stage one, the clear liquids diet. Thought to contain no fiber. Allowed on the low-fiber diet.

Histamine: Avoid.

Lectins: One source mentioned that supplements containing liquorice root help to heal a leaky gut. Another source mentioned that liquorice contains concentrated levels of lectins. Test carefully.

Oxalates: One that is potentially on your 'culprits' list. Extremely high; licorice root had a total oxalate concentration of 3569 mg per 100 g. (source: *Scientific Electronic Library of Brazil*).

Salicylates: Very high. In a 1985 analysis of salicylates contents of foods by Swain et al, licorice was found to contain a very high level of salicylates, about 10 times higher than peppermints which are considered problematic for those who are sensitive.

Lobster

- DASH: Fat: ✓ Sodium: ✗ Sugar: ✓
- Diverticulitis: Stage 1: ✗ Stage 2: ✓ Stage 3: ✗
- Histamine: ✗
- Lectin: ✓
- Oxalate: ✓
- Salicylates: ✓

DASH Diet (Hypertension): Watch the sodium here. Several sources seem to suggest lobster is allowed on the DASH diet. Avoid serving lobster with butter and eat in moderation. *Saturated fat content: 0.106g (per 100g), Sodium content: 700mg (per 100g), 30% daily value based on a 2,000 calorie diet, Sugar content: 0g (per 100g).*

Diverticulitis: No solid foods can be eaten at stage one, the clear liquids diet. Seafood contains no fiber, so lobster is allowed on the low-fiber diet.

Histamine: See notes under "Fish".

Lectins: Thought to be low in lectin.

Oxalates: See notes under "Fish".

Salicylates: Fish contains no to only trace amounts of salicylates, according to most reliable sources.

Loganberry

- DASH: Fat: ✓ Sodium: ✓ Sugar: ✗
- Diverticulitis: Stage 1: ✗ Stage 2: ✗ Stage 3: ✓
- Histamine: 😳
- Lectin: 😳
- Oxalate: 😳
- Salicylates: ✗

DASH Diet (Hypertension): Low in saturated fat and sodium content but high in sugar. Eat in moderation. *Saturated fat content: 0.3g (per 100g), Sodium content: 1mg (per 100g), less than 1% daily value based on a 2,000 calorie diet, Sugar content: 7.7g (per 100g)* (source: *Nutrition Value*).

Diverticulitis: No solid foods can be eaten at stage one, the clear liquids diet. Allowed on the high-fiber diet.

Histamine: Test carefully.

Lectins: A cross between raspberries and blackberries. As raspberries and blackberries are thought to contain moderate amounts of lectins, we think loganberries should be rated the same.

Oxalates: Many nutritional benefits; we have found it difficult to get reliable data on oxalate content. Test carefully.

Salicylates: Like most berries, loganberries are considered high in salicylates.

Lychee

- DASH: Fat: ✓ Sodium: ✓ Sugar: ✗
- Diverticulitis: Stage 1: ✗ Stage 2: ✓ Stage 3: ✗
- Histamine: ✓
- Lectin: ✗
- Oxalate: ✓
- Salicylates: ✗

Also known as *litchi*. According to the US Department of Agriculture, a cup of lychees contains almost 29 g of sugar. We therefore, suggest limiting lychee even if it's allowed on the diet. If choosing canned lychees, go for water-packed canned lychees and check the sugar content and avoid those with added sweeteners. Never eat unripe lychees. These are poisonous and can cause extremely low blood sugar (source: *CNN Health*).

DASH Diet (Hypertension): Low in saturated fat and sodium content but high in sugar. It's thought to contain potassium which helps to maintain blood pressure. Eat in moderation. *Saturated fat content: 0.1g (per 100g), Sodium content: 1mg (per 100g), less than 1% daily value based on a 2,000 calorie diet, Sugar content: 15g (per 100g).*

Diverticulitis: No solid foods can be eaten at stage one, the clear liquids diet. Low in fiber, so allowed on the low-fiber diet.

Histamine: Must be fresh, not canned.

Lectins: A study found lectins in the seeds of litchi fruits (source: *A glucose/mannose binding lectin from litchi (Litchi chinensis) seeds: Biochemical and biophysical characterizations*). Test carefully.

Oxalates: Less than 2 mg of oxalate per 100 grams (source: *UPMC*).

Salicylates: Fresh lychee is moderately high in salicylates with up to .49 mg per 100 g.

Macadamia

- DASH: Fat: ✗ Sodium: ✓ Sugar: ✓
- Diverticulitis: Stage 1: ✗ Stage 2: ✗ Stage 3: ✓
- Histamine: 😐
- Lectin: ✓
- Oxalate: ✗
- Salicylates: 😐

DASH Diet (Hypertension): Although macadamia nuts are high in saturated fats, like many nuts, they are rich in nutrients and antioxidants. Because of this, macadamia nuts can be included in the DASH diet in moderation. *Saturated fat content: 12g (per 100g), Sodium content: 5 mg (per 100g), less than 1% daily value based on a 2,000 calorie diet, Sugar content: 4.6g (per 100g).*

Diverticulitis: No solid foods can be eaten at stage one, the clear liquids diet. Allowed on the high-fiber diet.

Histamine: Test carefully.

Lectins: Tolerated.

Oxalates: Moderate to high, 10 – 25 mg per 100 grams (source: *https://www.thekidneydietitian.org/low-oxalate-nuts/*). See Nuts for more information.

Salicylates: Macadamia nuts have a moderately high level of salicylates with just over .50 mg per 100 g however, some people have reported tolerating them in small amounts.

Malt

- DASH: Fat: ✗ Sodium: ✓ Sugar: ✗
- Diverticulitis: Stage 1: ✗ Stage 2: ✗ Stage 3: ✓
- Histamine: ✗
- Lectin: ✗
- Oxalate: ✗
- Salicylates: ✓

Malt is a cereal grain that has been dried in a process called malting. Malt is often used in making beer, liquor, baked goods and desserts (source: *Food52*).

DASH Diet (Hypertension): Limit your malt intake as it is higher in saturated fat and sugars.

Diverticulitis: No solid foods can be eaten at stage one, the clear liquids diet. Allowed on the high-fiber diet.

Histamine: Includes barley malt and malt extract . Avoid.

Lectins: Avoid barley malt as barley is high in lectins.

Oxalates: High, best avoided.

Salicylates: The germinated cereal grain dried in a process called "malting" is low in salicylates, but if you're on a gluten-free diet, you'll want to avoid it.

Malt extract

- DASH: Fat: ✓ Sodium: Not specified Sugar: ✗
- Diverticulitis: Stage 1: ✗ Stage 2: ✗ Stage 3: ✓
- Histamine: ✗
- Lectin: ✗
- Oxalate: ✗
- Salicylates: ✓

Malt may be further processed to form malt extract (source: *Briess*). It's thought to be high in antioxidants.

DASH Diet (Hypertension): It's thought to be high in sugar, so best to avoid it.

Diverticulitis: No solid foods can be eaten at stage one, the clear liquids diet. Allowed on the high-fiber diet.

Histamine: Avoid.

Lectins: Derived from barley grains. Avoid as barley is high in lectins.

Oxalates: High, best avoided.

Salicylates: A rich source of soluble fiber, malt extract is also low in salicylates.

Maltodextrin

- DASH: Fat: ✓ Sodium: ✓ Sugar: ✗
- Diverticulitis: Stage 1: ✗ Stage 2: ✗ Stage 3: ✓
- Histamine: 😕
- Lectin: ✗
- Oxalate: 😕
- Salicylates: 😕

A highly processed form of carbohydrate that's extracted from corn, rice, potato and other plants. It's commonly found in artificial sweeteners, yogurt, beer, baked goods and nutrition bars, to name a few (source: *Medicine Net*). Used to thicken foods and liquids, improve texture, flavor and increase shelf life, maltodextrin has no nutritional value (source: *Medical News Today*).

DASH Diet (Hypertension): As it's a powder typically found in processed foods, it's best to avoid it.

Diverticulitis: Maltodextrin is used as a type of fiber in food additives.

Histamine: Quite a considerable difference between major experts about whether maltodextrin is good for those who are histamine intolerant. Approach cautiously. While maltodextrin on its own may be lower histamine, the result may be higher histamine levels in the body. Check out 'sweeteners' for better natural alternatives.

Lectins: Highly processed and high in lectins. Not an ingredient we like. One to put on your 'avoid' list.

Oxalates: See "sweeteners". Maltodextrin is often avoided by those looking to optimize a natural diet as it can be GMO and corn-derived.

Salicylates: Not the best choice for those following a more natural, whole food diet as it's often derived from GMO corn, though it is typically low in salicylates. See "sweeteners".

Mandarin orange

- DASH: Fat: ✓ Sodium: ✓ Sugar: ✗
- Diverticulitis: Stage 1: ✗ Stage 2: ✗ Stage 3: ✓
- Histamine: ✗
- Lectin: 😕
- Oxalate: ✗
- Salicylates: ✗

DASH Diet (Hypertension): Although mandarin oranges are high in sugar, they have many health benefits that may make them worthwhile to include in your diet. Mandarin oranges are loaded with fiber and potassium, which help lower blood pressure (source: *WebMD*).

Diverticulitis: No solid foods can be eaten at stage one, the clear liquids diet. Allowed on the high-fiber diet.

Histamine: see "citrus fruit"

Lectins: Opinion is split. One source confirmed oranges are a source of lectins. However, another source noted oranges contain D-Mannose, a powerful natural lectin-blocker. Test carefully.

Oxalates: 10 – 25 mg per 100 grams/ml, both for the fruit and the juice, this makes it moderately high in oxalates (source: *UPMC*) and high on our list.

Salicylates: Fresh mandarin is moderately high in salicylates with potentially over .5 mg. As with everything on a low-salicylate diet, proceed with caution and test carefully first.

Mango

- DASH: Fat: ✔ Sodium: ✔ Sugar: ✗
- Diverticulitis: Stage 1: ✗ Stage 2: ✗ Stage 3: ✔
- Histamine: 😐
- Lectin: ✔
- Oxalate: ✗
- Salicylates: 😐

DASH Diet (Hypertension): Mangoes are a higher sugar fruit, but can be eaten in moderation as part of a healthy diet. *Saturated fat content: 0.1g (per 100g), Sodium content: 1 mg (per 100g) less than 1% daily value based on a 2,000 calorie diet, Sugar content: 14g (per 100g).*

Diverticulitis: No solid foods can be eaten at stage one, the clear liquids diet. Allowed on the high-fiber diet.

Histamine: Test carefully.

Lectins: Tolerated on a low lectin diet however, we believe a lower sugar diet is better for overall health, therefore limiting ripe mangoes due to their high sugar levels.

Oxalates: 10 - 25mg per 100 grams, moderate (source: *UPMC*). Based on this and other food lists such as the Urinary Stones site, we consider this moderate to high.

Salicylates: Opinion varies between the major sites. Proceed with caution if you are highly sensitive. While high in vitamins A and C, it also contains a high level of natural fruit sugars.

Maple syrup

- DASH: Fat: ✔ Sodium: ✔ Sugar: ✗
- Diverticulitis: Stage 1: ✔ Stage 2: ✔ Stage 3: ✗
- Histamine: ✔
- Lectin: ✗
- Oxalate: 😐
- Salicylates: ✔

DASH Diet (Hypertension): Although high in sugar, some recommend the DASH diet include real maple syrup as a healthy sweet treat replacement. (Source: *Winchester Hospital*). *Saturated fat content: 0g (per 100g), Sodium content: 12mg (per 100g) less than 1% daily value based on a 2,000 calorie diet, Sugar content: 68g (per 100g).*

Diverticulitis: Allowed at stages one and two, but it is thought to contain no fiber and eating too much of it could cause a spike in your blood sugar levels and insulin (source: *Cleveland Clinic*).

Histamine: Note previous comments about lowering sugar levels for optimum health in relation to histamine intolerance.

Lectins: Because of the higher sugar content, maple syrup should be avoided. Yacon syrup has been recommended instead.

Oxalates: Note previous comments about keeping sugar levels low for optimum health regardless of oxalate levels.

Salicylates: Thought to be low in salicylates (but high in sugar).

Margarine

- DASH: Fat: ✗ Sodium: ✔ Sugar: ✔

- Diverticulitis: Stage 1: ✗ Stage 2: ✓ Stage 3: ✗
- Histamine: ✗
- Lectin: ✗
- Oxalate: ✓
- Salicylates: ✗

DASH Diet (Hypertension): Margarine is typically limited in the DASH diet due to its high saturated fat content. *Saturated fat content: 15g (per 100g), Sodium content: 2mg (per 100g) less than 1% daily value based on a 2,000 calorie diet, Sugar content: 0g.*

Diverticulitis: Margarine contains no fiber. Allowed on the low-fiber diet.

Histamine: Almost always contains sub-optimal ingredients.

Lectins: A processed food - thought to be high in lectins.

Oxalates: Low. However, not always a brilliant choice for general health because of the added preservatives.

Salicylates: Margarine and salicylates is a complicated relationship. As with other intolerances such as histamine intolerance, some foods contain salicylate, and some foods cause a salicylate reaction. Margarine falls in that category. We can't vouch for the exact levels of salicylates in individual margarine, however, margarine is thought to contain preservatives that can mimic salicylates or cause salicylate flare-ups. This is besides trans fats, which are associated with an increased risk of heart disease.

Marrow

- DASH:
  - Bone marrow: Fat: ✗ Sodium: N/A Sugar: N/A
  - Vegetable marrow: Fat: ✓ Sodium: N/A Sugar: N/A

- Diverticulitis: Stage 1: ✗ Stage 2: ✗ Stage 3: ✓
- Histamine: ✓
- Lectin: ✗
- Oxalate: ✓
- Salicylates: 🤷

DASH Diet (Hypertension): The sodium and sugar content of marrow is unknown. Avoid bone marrow as this is thought to be high in saturated fat content and high in calories. **Bone marrow**: *Saturated fat content: 84.4g (per 100g)* (source: *Fatsecret Platform API*). **Vegetable marrow**: *Saturated fat content: 0.5g (per 100g).*

Diverticulitis: No solid foods can be eaten at stage one, the clear liquids diet. Allowed on the high-fiber diet.

Histamine: Tolerated.

Lectins: Thought to be a source of lectins, as are courgettes (see courgette). Removing the seeds may help lower the lectin content, which is easier with a marrow than a courgette.

Oxalates: Low.

Salicylates: Marrow ranges from low to moderate depending on the source, containing over .15 mg per 100g. As it is categorized as moderate by some reliable sources, it's best to proceed with caution.

Mascarpone cheese

- DASH: Fat: ✗ Sodium: ✓ Sugar: ✓

- Diverticulitis: Stage 1: ✗ Stage 2: ✓ Stage 3: ✗
- Histamine: 😕
- Lectin: 😕
- Oxalate: ✓
- Salicylates: ✓

A type of soft Italian cream cheese.

DASH Diet (Hypertension): High in saturated fat, so try to avoid on the DASH diet. *Saturated fat content: 30g (per 100g), Sodium content: 33mg (per 100g), 2% daily value based on a 2,000 calorie diet, Sugar content: 3.3g (per 100g)* (source: *Eat This Much*).

Diverticulitis: No solid foods can be eaten at stage one, the clear liquids diet. Cheese contains no fiber so they're allowed on the low-fiber diet.

Histamine: See other comments about soft cheeses. May be better tolerated than hard cheeses.

Lectins: Some sources claim that very high fat dairy products such as cream cheeses are low in casein and therefore low in lectin. Other sources mention all dairy products contain casein and should be avoided. Test carefully.

Oxalates: See other comments under Cheeses.

Salicylates: Most cheeses are thought to be very low in salicylates.
Choose mascarpone made from 100 percent grass-fed animals for the highest level of nutrients and avoid processed types which may contain salicylates along with other potentially harmful ingredients.

Mate tea

- DASH: Fat: ✓ Sodium: ✓ Sugar: ✓
- Diverticulitis: Stage 1: ✓ Stage 2: ✓ Stage 3: ✗
- Histamine: ✗
- Lectin: ✓
- Oxalate: ✗
- Salicylates: ✗

Mate tea is thought to help with several conditions such as headaches and depression (source: *Mayo Clinic*). It's high in antioxidants and a source of caffeine.

DASH Diet (Hypertension): Watch your intake as too much caffeine could increase blood pressure. *Saturated fat content: 0g (per tea bag, 3g), Sodium content: 0mg (per tea bag, 3g), Sugar content: 0g (per tea bag, 3g)* (source: *Fatsecret Platform API*).

Diverticulitis: Tea with no milk or cream is allowed at stage one, the clear liquid diet. Also allowed on the low-fiber diet.

Histamine: The Histamine Intolerance Awareness Site lists mate tea under '*foods that have been reported to block the diamine oxidase (DAO) enzyme*'

Lectins: It's thought that tea is allowed on a low-lectin diet.

Oxalates: Contains a moderate amount of oxalates.

Salicylates: Mate, like most teas, is high in salicylates.

Melon

- DASH: Fat: ✓ Sodium: ✓ Sugar: ✗
- Diverticulitis: Stage 1: ✗ Stage 2: ✓ Stage 3: ✗
- Histamine: ✓
- Lectin: ✗
- Oxalate: ✓
- Salicylates: ✗

DASH Diet (Hypertension): Fruits like melon can be eaten on the DASH diet to replace more unhealthy sweets. Try a fruit cup to appease your sweet tooth. *Saturated fat content: 0.1g (per 100g), Sodium content: 16mg (per 100g), less than 1% daily value based on a 2,000 calorie diet, Sugar content: 8g (per 100g).*

Diverticulitis: No solid foods can be eaten at stage one, the clear liquids diet. Low in fiber, so allowed on the low-fiber diet.

Histamine: The Histamine Intolerance Site lists melon as low histamine, but please note that watermelon is listed in a different category as medium histamine and should be approached with caution.

Lectins: High in lectins. One to put on your 'avoid' list.

Oxalates: Cantaloupe, honeydew, and watermelon are all thought to be low in oxalate, which is excellent news. A good fruit choice.

Salicylates: It all depends on what type of melon. The salicylates in this fruit depend on the type of melon, with most containing a moderate to a high amount. Watermelon was analyzed to contain moderate amounts of salicylates, while other melons, such as cantaloupe (also known as *rock-melon*), were shown to have a much higher level.

Milk

- DASH: Fat: ✓ Sodium: ✓ Sugar: ✓
- Diverticulitis: Stage 1: ✗ Stage 2: ✓ Stage 3: ✗
- Histamine: ✓
- Lectin: 🤔
- Oxalate: ✓
- Salicylates: ✓

Dairy is a great source of protein and calcium.

DASH Diet (Hypertension): Allowed. Opt for fat-free or low-fat milk for the best DASH diet choice (source: Winchester Hospital). *Saturated fat content: 0.6g (per 100g), Sodium content: 44 mg (per 100g) 1% daily value based on a 2,000 calorie diet, Sugar content: 5g (per 100g).*

Diverticulitis: Avoid at stage one the clear liquid diet as milk causes flare-ups. All liquids should be clear. Milk contains no fiber, so they're allowed on a low-fiber diet.

Histamine: Includes UHT, pasteurized. Milk powder and lactose-free milk may be higher in histamine.

Lectins: Goat and sheep milk are acceptable on a low-lectin diet. As for cow's milk. It depends on the type. Certain kinds of milk are high in A1 casein, which can be high in lectins. It's thought that milk from cows that originated in the Channel Islands and Southern France are better on a low-lectin diet. Test store-bought milk carefully.

Oxalates: Many on a low-oxalate diet seek more calcium. The University of Virginia Digestive Health Center notes: "*Eat plenty of calcium-rich foods. Calcium binds to oxalate so that it isn't absorbed into your blood and cannot reach your kidneys. Dairy is free of oxalate and high in calcium, so it is an ideal choice. Choose skim, low fat, or full fat* versions depending on your weight goals. If you are lactose intolerant, look for lactose-free dairy such as Lactaid brand, or eat yogurt or kefir instead." The respected Dr. Jockers says this about dairy products: *"Dairy: Most food sources contain little to no oxalates. Examples include eggs, cheeses, yogurt, and plain milk (chocolate is a source of oxalates so stray from the chocolate milk)."*

Salicylates: Most dairy products typically have little or no salicylates, including animal milk of all types like goat's and cow's milk. Important note: Be aware that non-animal milk often used in trendy coffee shops like almond and coconut milk, has high salicylates.

Millet

- DASH: Fat: ✓ Sodium: ✓ Sugar: ✓
- Diverticulitis: Stage 1: ✗ Stage 2: ✗ Stage 3: ✓
- Histamine: ✓
- Lectin: ✓
- Oxalate: ✗
- Salicylates: ✓

Millet is a healthy grain option to include in your diet.

DASH Diet (Hypertension): Allowed. *Saturated fat content: 0.5g (per 100g), Sodium content: 4 mg (per 100g) less than 1% daily value based on a 2,000 calorie diet, Sugar content: 1.7g (per 100g).*

Diverticulitis: No solid foods can be eaten at stage one, the clear liquids diet. Allowed on the high-fiber diet.

Histamine: Tolerated.

Lectins: A lectin-free grain and high in antioxidants. Tolerated on a low-lectin diet.

Oxalates: The grain is very high, with over 15 mg of oxalate per 100 g. According to a study by the Cereals and Grains Association, *"The levels of total oxalate in raw cereals and millets varied between 3.6 and 20.0 mg/100 g, and in cooked cereals and millets it ranged from 2.4 mg/100 g in rice to 13.4 mg/100 g in pearl millet... The levels of soluble oxalate in raw cereals and millets ranged from 1.9 to 9.1 mg/100 g."*

Salicylates: Millet contains negligible amounts of salicylates.

Minced meat

- DASH: Fat: ✗ Sodium: ✓ Sugar: ✓
- Diverticulitis: Stage 1: ✗ Stage 2: ✓ Stage 3: ✗
- Histamine: Fresh: ✓ Open sale: 😖
- Lectin: ✓
- Oxalate: ✓
- Salicylates: ✗

DASH Diet (Hypertension): Minced meat is high in saturated fat. Try to avoid it. *Saturated fat content: 11g (per 100g), Sodium content: 67mg (per 100g), 2% daily value based on a 2,000 calorie diet, Sugar content: 0g (per 100g).*

Diverticulitis: No solid foods can be eaten at stage one, the clear liquids diet. Meat contains no fiber, so minced meat is allowed on the low-fiber diet.

Histamine: If eaten immediately after its production, minced meat is allowed. However - and this is a big one - if it is left then it can rise in histamine quicker than other forms of meat. Some histamine-intolerant people even buy their own mincer to avoid this issue. If you are not quite that committed yet (and we don't blame you if you aren't!), then look for the freshest mince with the longest best before date, and eat immediately or freeze. We have given this one two emojis, one for completely freshly ground and one for open sale, as it's hard to know each portion's freshness and histamine levels.

Lectins: Avoid corn-fed minced meat and opt for grass-fed instead.

Oxalates: Low oxalate. However, eating large portions of meat can potentially increase the risk of kidney stones.

Salicylates: Minced meat may contain some beef which is typically salicylate free, but it's generally a mixture of ingredients that are high in salicylates, such as spices, dried fruit, and distilled spirits.

Mint

- DASH: Fat: ✓ Sodium: ✓ Sugar: ✓
- Diverticulitis: Stage 1: 😷 Stage 2: ✓ Stage 3: ✗
- Histamine: ✓
- Lectin: ✓
- Oxalate: 😷
- Salicylates: ✗

DASH Diet (Hypertension): Allowed. Use mint to spruce up dishes, or drink it as a tea. *Saturated fat content: 0.2g (per 100g), Sodium content: 31 mg (per 100mg), 1% daily value based on a 2,000 calorie diet, Sugar content: 0g (per 100g).*

Diverticulitis: Mint tea with no milk or cream is allowed at stage one, the clear liquid diet. Low in fiber so allowed on the low-fiber diet.

Histamine: Tolerated.

Lectins: Thought to be low-lectin.

Oxalates: Mint tea is low in oxalates. Spearmint is moderate.

Salicylates: Mint, whether the herb, peppermint candy or in chewing gum, is high in salicylates.

Morel

- DASH: Fat: ✓ Sodium: ✓ Sugar: ✓
- Diverticulitis: Stage 1: ✗ Stage 2: 😷 Stage 3: ✓
- Histamine: ✗
- Lectin: ✓
- Oxalate: ✗
- Salicylates: 😷

DASH Diet (Hypertension): Allowed. *Saturated fat content: 0.1g (per 100g), Sodium content: 21mg (per 100g) 1% daily value based on a 2,000 calorie diet, Sugar content: 0.6g (per 100g).*

Diverticulitis: No solid foods can be eaten at stage one, the clear liquids diet. Whilst this mushroom doesn't contain the highest amounts of fiber compared to other veg, it can still be eaten on the high-fiber diet. Test carefully on a low-fiber diet.

Histamine: Avoid.

Lectins: A type of wild mushroom that's difficult to find (source: *Wild Food UK*). As these are rare, they tend to be expensive and used in gourmet meals. Given that most mushrooms contain relatively low lectin, morels should be the same too.

Oxalates: Low.

Salicylates: There is no information on the content of salicylates in morel or truffles that we could find, making it impossible to categorize it accurately. Fresh mushrooms have a low level at about .24 mg per 100 g, which may be a sign but proceed with caution if you're sensitive.

Morello cherries

- DASH: Fat: ✓ Sodium: ✓ Sugar: ✗
- Diverticulitis: Stage 1: ✗ Stage 2: ✗ Stage 3: ✓
- Histamine: ✓
- Lectin: ✓
- Oxalate: ✓
- Salicylates: ✓

Morello cherries are tart, sour cherries that are most often consumed dried, frozen, or juiced. Morello cherries contain 20 times more vitamin A than sweet cherries (source: *Healthline*).

DASH Diet (Hypertension): Watch the sugar content. *Saturated fat content: 0g (per 100g), Sodium content: 7.4mg (per 100g), 1% daily value based on a 2,000 calorie diet, Sugar content: 8.49g (per 100g)* (source: *Eat This Much, Fatsecret Platform API*).

Diverticulitis: No solid foods can be eaten at stage one, the clear liquids diet. Allowed on the high-fiber diet.

Histamine: See other comments on 'Cherry' and 'Acerola'.

Lectins: Given that morello cherries are a type of cherry, they should be low in lectins. Test carefully.

Oxalates: Cherries are considered low in oxalate with around 2 mg per 100 grams (source: *UPMC*). Canned Morello cherries are considered be high in salicylates, a naturally occurring compound in plants.

Salicylates: Sour canned morello cherries have a low amount of salicylates at less than .25 mg per 100 mg.

Mozzarella cheese

- DASH: Fat: ✗ Sodium: ✓ Sugar: ✓
- Diverticulitis: Stage 1: ✗ Stage 2: ✓ Stage 3: ✗
- Histamine: 🤔
- Lectin: 🤔
- Oxalate: ✓
- Salicylates: ✓

DASH Diet (Hypertension): Mozzarella cheese is high in saturated fat, so try to limit or avoid on the DASH diet. *Saturated fat content: 11g (per 100g), Sodium content: 16 mg (per 100g) less than 1% daily value based on a 2,000 calorie diet, Sugar content: 1.2g (per 100g).*

Diverticulitis: No solid foods can be eaten at stage one, the clear liquids diet. Cheese contains no fiber, so they're allowed on a low-fiber diet.

Histamine: See other comments on soft cheeses. Mozzarella is often well tolerated by many who are histamine intolerant but not everybody. Soft cheeses are a better option than hard cheese or moldy cheese.

Lectins: Mozzarella is thought to contain less casein protein than hard cheeses. Test carefully.

Oxalates: See other comments on soft cheeses.

Salicylates: *"Most cheeses are thought to be very low in salicylates.*

Choose cheeses made from 100 percent grass-fed animals for the highest level of nutrients and avoid processed types which may contain salicylates along with other potentially harmful ingredients."

Mulberry

- DASH: Fat: ✔ Sodium: ✔ Sugar: ✘
- Diverticulitis: Stage 1: ✘ Stage 2: ✘ Stage 3: ✔
- Histamine: 😐
- Lectin: ✘
- Oxalate: ✘
- Salicylates: ✘

Mulberries contain loads of heart-healthy antioxidants.

DASH Diet (Hypertension): Although they have higher sugar content, mulberries can be part of a healthy diet in moderation. *Saturated fat content: 0g (per 100g), Sodium content: 10 mg (per 100g) less than 1% daily value based on a 2,000 calorie diet, Sugar content: 8g.*

Diverticulitis: No solid foods can be eaten at stage one, the clear liquids diet. Allowed on the high-fiber diet.

Histamine: Test carefully.

Lectins: A rich source of lectins (source: *Saeed B, Baranwal VK, Khurana P. Identification and Expression Profiling of the Lectin Gene Superfamily in Mulberry*). One to put on your 'avoid' list.

Oxalates: Calcium oxalate crystals are found in mulberry leaves.

Salicylates: As a berry, mulberries have a high level of salicylates with .76 mg per 100 g.

Mung beans (germinated, sprouting)

- DASH: Fat: ✔ Sodium: ✔ Sugar: ✘
- Diverticulitis: Stage 1: ✘ Stage 2: ✘ Stage 3: ✔
- Histamine: 😐
- Lectin: ✘
- Oxalate: ✘
- Salicylates: ✔

Mung beans are part of the legume family.

DASH Diet (Hypertension): Packed with protein, fiber, and antioxidants, mung beans can be a great addition to a healthy diet (source: *Holland and Barrett*). *Saturated fat content: 0.3g (per 100g), Sodium content: 15 mg (per 100g), less than 1% daily value based on a 2,000 calorie diet, Sugar content: 7g (per 100g).*

Diverticulitis: No solid foods can be eaten at stage one, the clear liquids diet. Allowed on the high-fiber diet.

Histamine: Test carefully.

Lectins: A source of lectins, although lectin content is reduced significantly after the sprouting process (source: *Superfood Evolution*). Sprouting can be done at home by following the process: *"1) Soak legumes to soften, 2) rinse well with cool water, 3) drain water from the jar 4) Repeat steps 2 and 3 until sprouts form and 5) Store in the fridge until ready to eat."* (source: *Live Eat Learn*). Avoid eating mung bean sprouts raw.

Oxalates: Moderate in oxalates, with around 8 mg of oxalate per half a cup (source: *St. Joseph's Healthcare Hamilton*).

Salicylates: Mungbeans are free of salicylates.

Mushrooms, different types

- DASH: Fat: ✓ Sodium: ✓ Sugar: ✓
- Diverticulitis: Stage 1: ✗ Stage 2: 😐 Stage 3: ✓
- Histamine: 😐
- Lectin: ✓
- Oxalate: ✓
- Salicylates: ✓

DASH Diet (Hypertension): Allowed. Mushrooms are a versatile food that can be incorporated into various dishes. *Saturated fat content: 0.1g (per 100g), Sodium content: 5 mg (per 100g), less than 1% daily value based on a 2,000 calorie diet, Sugar content: 2g (per 100g).*

Diverticulitis: No solid foods can be eaten at stage one, the clear liquids diet. Whilst mushroom doesn't contain the highest amounts of fiber compared to other veg, they can still be eaten on a high-fiber diet. Test carefully on a low-fiber diet.

Histamine: Another ingredient where opinion is divided. Please test carefully.

Lectins: Mushrooms fall under the lowest lectin content options for a low-lectin diet.

Oxalates: Low oxalate, but thoughts vary on how much and the type of mushroom. The University of Chicago suggests little or no oxalates in mushrooms. Listed as 'Safe To Eat' on the Unusual Ingredients website.

Salicylates: Mushrooms of all types have a low amount of salicylates, with analysis showing a range of up to but not over .25 g per 100 g.

Mustard and mustard seeds

- DASH: Fat: ✓ Sodium: ✗ Sugar: ✓
- Diverticulitis: Stage 1: ✗ Stage 2: ✗ Stage 3: ✓
- Histamine: ✗
- Lectin: ✓
- Oxalate: ✓
- Salicylates: ✗

DASH Diet (Hypertension): Mustard is high in sodium. Try to avoid or limit.

Diverticulitis: No solid foods can be eaten at stage one, the clear liquids diet. Mustard and mustard seeds are high in fiber.

Histamine: Avoid.

Lectins: Tolerated on a low-lectin diet.

Oxalates: With just 0.1 - 2.9 mg per 100 g (source: *Low Oxalate Diet - Mark O'Brien MD*), all mustard is very low in oxalate, including our favorite, Dijon.

Salicylates: Mustard and mustard seeds are very high in salicylates.

Napa cabbage

- DASH: Fat: ✓ Sodium: ✓ Sugar: ✓

- Diverticulitis: Stage 1: ✗ Stage 2: ✓ Stage 3: ✓
- Histamine: ✓
- Lectin: ✓
- Oxalate: ✓
- Salicylates: ✓

Also known as *Chinese Cabbage*. Falls under the cruciferous vegetable family (includes broccoli, kale, Brussel sprouts, radish etc.), and it's often used in dishes such as stir-fry.

DASH Diet (Hypertension): Allowed. *Saturated fat content: 0g (per 100g), Sodium content: 11mg (per 100g), less than 1% daily value based on a 2,000 calorie diet, Sugar content: 0g (per 100g).*

Diverticulitis: No solid foods can be eaten at stage one, the clear liquids diet. Low in fiber. Whilst this cabbage doesn't contain the highest amounts of fiber compared to other veg, it can still be eaten on a high-fiber diet.

Histamine: Tolerated.

Lectins: Thought to be low-lectin and rich in vitamin C, folate and fiber.

Oxalates: We love cabbage. It's very versatile and cheap, even organic. It is thought to be very low in oxalates along with similar veggies like endive, cabbage, and lettuce.

Salicylates: Thankfully, cabbage is considered low in salicylates and versatile and cheap, even when purchasing organic. Plus, just a half-cup cooked provides about a third of your daily vitamin C requirements.

Nectarine

- DASH: Fat: ✓ Sodium: ✓ Sugar: ✗
- Diverticulitis: Stage 1: ✗ Stage 2: ✓ Stage 3: ✓
- Histamine: 🤔
- Lectin: ✓
- Oxalate: ✓
- Salicylates: ✗

DASH Diet (Hypertension): Nectarines are high in sugar but can be included in moderation as part of a healthy diet. *Saturated fat content: 0g (per 100g), Sodium content: 0mg (per 100g), 0% daily value based on a 2,000 calorie diet, Sugar content: 8g (per 100g).*

Diverticulitis: No solid foods can be eaten at stage one, the clear liquids diet. Allowed on the low-fiber diet if unripe and no skin.

Histamine: This is one where opinion varies. On SIGHI, it is ranked as low histamine. On the respected site SFGATE it is noted as high histamine. And the Histamine Intolerance Site sensibly comes down in the middle. Test carefully.

Lectins: Best to consume when nectarine is in season. As with other fruits, when in season, it may contain fewer lectins than when they're out of season.

Oxalates: It's thought to contain little to no oxalates.

Salicylates: Nectarine is another fruit that is quite high in salicylates. Not all sources agree on the exact levels, but they tend to agree that this is a fruit to approach with caution.

Nettle tea

- DASH: Fat: ✓ Sodium: ✓ Sugar: ✓

- Diverticulitis: Stage 1: ✓ Stage 2: ✓ Stage 3: ✗
- Histamine: ✗
- Lectin: ✗
- Oxalate: 😐
- Salicylates: 😐

Nettle tea is made by infusing a stinging nettle plant in hot water. It is rich in antioxidants (source: *Medical News Today*).

DASH Diet (Hypertension): Allowed. *Saturated fat content: 0g (per 100g), Sodium content: 0g (per 100g), 0% daily value based on a 2,000 calorie diet, Sugar content: 0g (per 100g).*

Diverticulitis: Tea with no milk or cream is allowed at stage one, the clear liquid diet. Also allowed on the low-fiber diet.

Histamine: Alison Vickery quotes excellent studies which suggest nettle is a potent antihistamine (working at the H1 receptor) and mast cell stabilizer. So this may be a good option. However, approach cautiously as some still react to nettle tea.

Lectins: A study found "unusual" lectins in stinging nettles (source: *Science Direct: An unusual lectin from stinging nettle (Urtica dioica) rhizomes*). Best to avoid.

Oxalates: Young leaves are not thought to have much oxalate. Research before you consume nettles or nettle tea. Go slowly and carefully. The website KidneySchool notes: *"If you make tea out of fresh nettle leaves, use small, young leaves. Older nettle leaves can contain oxalate, which can irritate the kidneys."* Research on PubMed suggests nettles may be good for kidney stones: *"Urtica dioica or "Stinging Nettle", which belongs to the nettle genus of the Urticaceae family, is used as tea in Austrian medicine. It has shown a long history of beneficial therapeutic effects toward urinary ailments, specifically with the urinary tract and kidney stones. Its major bioactive phytochemicals include flavonoids, anthocyanins, and saponins. These phytoconstituents provide the possibility of inhibition of calcium and oxalate deposition and crystals growth."* Zhang H., Li N., Li K., Li P.

Salicylates: There have not been many studies looking at the amount of salicylates in nettle leaves, although some reports indicate that it is very low. Frustratingly, as we cannot be sure, we've ranked it in the middle, meaning consume a small amount until you know how it will affect you. This is one of the foods and ingredients we hope to update on this list as more research becomes available.

Nori seaweed

- DASH: Fat: ✓ Sodium: ✓ Sugar: ✓
- Diverticulitis: Stage 1: ✗ Stage 2: ✗ Stage 3: ✓
- Histamine: ✗
- Lectin: ✓
- Oxalate: ✓
- Salicylates: ✗

DASH Diet (Hypertension): Allowed. Nori seaweed boasts many health benefits, such as supporting heart health, boosting the immune system, and balancing blood sugar levels (source: *BBC Good Food*). *Saturated fat content: 0.1g (per 100g), Sodium content: 48mg (per 100g), 2% daily value based on a 2,000 calorie diet, Sugar content: 0.5g (per 100g).*

Diverticulitis: No solid foods can be eaten at stage one, the clear liquids diet. Allowed on the high-fiber diet.

Histamine: Avoid.

Lectins: Acceptable.

Oxalates: Might help prevent kidney stones. Best consumed in moderation because it has very high iodine levels.

Salicylates: Seaweed, including Nori seaweed, is very high in salicylates.

Nutmeg
- DASH: Fat: ✗ Sodium: ✓ Sugar: ✓
- Diverticulitis: Stage 1: ✗ Stage 2: ✗ Stage 3: ✓
- Histamine: 😐
- Lectin: 😐
- Oxalate: ✓
- Salicylates: ✗

DASH Diet (Hypertension): Avoid eating large amounts of nutmeg as it is high in saturated fat. *Saturated fat content: 26g (per 100g), Sodium content: 16 mg (per 100g) less than 1% daily value based on a 2,000 calorie diet, Sugar content: 28g (per 100g).*

Diverticulitis: No solid foods can be eaten at stage one, the clear liquids diet. Allowed on the high-fiber diet.

Histamine: Nutmeg flower and nutmeg flower oil seem to be tolerated more effectively.

Lectins: Contains some lectins. Test carefully.

Oxalates: Thought to be low. Helen O'Connor, MS, RD lists this as containing 0-2mg of oxalates per serving.

Salicylates: Very high in salicylates as with most spices, nutmeg has been analyzed to contain 2.4 mg per 100 g. As with most spices, you may not be consuming many grams of nutmeg, but proceed with caution.

Nuts (see individual nuts for more details)
- DASH: Fat: ✗ Sodium: ✓ Sugar: ✓
- Diverticulitis: Stage 1: ✗ Stage 2: ✗ Stage 3: ✓
- Histamine: 😐
- Lectin: 😐
- Oxalate: ✗
- Salicylates: 😐

DASH Diet (Hypertension): Nuts are a vital part of the DASH diet. They add protein and healthy fat to your diet. They can be high in saturated fat, so eat in moderation. *Saturated fat content: 9g (per 100g), Sodium content: 273mg (per 100g) 11% daily value based on a 2,000 calorie diet, Sugar content: 4.2 g (per 100g).*

Diverticulitis: No solid foods can be eaten at stage one, the clear liquids diet. Allowed on the high-fiber diet.

Histamine: Nuts hugely depend, both from nut to nut, and on each individual batch in terms of freshness. One thing we consistently find with nuts is that the lower our histamine levels are, the more we can tolerate them. Conversely, if we are in the middle of a flare-up, we avoid nuts as bitter experience has shown that it causes more of a reaction. So please check each individual nut to see if it is listed in more detail.

Lectins: Depends on the type of nut. For example, cashew and peanuts are high in lectins. Check individual nuts in this food list.

Oxalates: Some say all nuts should be avoided on a Low-Oxalate diet. Check each individual nut. Almonds and Brazil nuts are thought to be high. The website Kidney Dietitian notes; *"Nuts & seeds are often taboo on a low oxalate, kidney stone friendly diet. This is probably because nuts and seeds are notorious for being high in oxalate. But, there are huge differences in oxalate between different nuts and seeds. If done correctly, nuts and seeds can be a part of a healthy low oxalate diet!"*

Salicylates: Check individual nuts in this food list. They can be very low or high, depending on the particular type.

Oats

- DASH: Fat: ✓ Sodium: ✓ Sugar: ✓
- Diverticulitis: Stage 1: ✗ Stage 2: ✗ Stage 3: ✓
- Histamine: ✓
- Lectin: ✗
- Oxalate: ✓
- Salicylates: ✓

DASH Diet (Hypertension): Allowed. Incorporate oats into your diet to add some healthy whole grains. *Saturated fat content: 0.2g (per 100g), Sodium content: 49mg (per 100g), 2% daily value based on a 2,000 calorie diet, Sugar content: 0.5g (per 100g).*

Diverticulitis: No solid foods can be eaten at stage one, the clear liquids diet. Allowed on the high-fiber diet.

Histamine: Oats are a real staple for those with histamine intolerance. But what about other oat products? Oat milk can be a good option when out and about and ordering coffee, for example. But always be mindful of other ingredients in oat drinks. For instance, several oat milks have many additives, whereas others only have three or four ingredients. So pick a good one - organic if possible.

Lectins: Oats are considered high in lectins and a major culprit for those on a low lectin diet. Consider sprouted oats instead, as these contain fewer lectins and should digest better. The sprouting process is thought to reduce the lectin content and make them easier to digest. Also, it's thought by some that cooking oats also reduces the lectin content.

Oxalates: Low. Making oats with milk instead of water is another way of increasing calcium.

Salicylates: Oats contain negligible amounts of salicylates if any.

Olive oil

- DASH: Fat: ✗ Sodium: ✓ Sugar: ✓
- Diverticulitis: Stage 1: ✗ Stage 2: ✓ Stage 3: ✗
- Histamine: ✓
- Lectin: ✓
- Oxalate: ✓
- Salicylates: ✗

DASH Diet (Hypertension): Olive oil is a healthy source of fat in the DASH diet. Eat in moderation. *Saturated fat content: 14g (per 100g), Sodium content: 2mg (per 100g), less than 1% daily value based on a 2,000 calorie diet, Sugar content: 0g (per 100g).*

Diverticulitis: Low in fiber, so allowed on the low-fiber diet.

Histamine: We believe a better choice when extra virgin. Organic extra virgin olive oil (or Organic EVOO as we like to call it) is even better.

Lectins: A source confirms that olive oil is acceptable on the lectin-free diet. The Woodland Institute notes that olive oil contains some lectins, but as they're full of antioxidants and healthy monounsaturated fats, the benefits outweigh the negatives. It's thought that they can be eaten without restriction, and it's unnecessary to eliminate them from your diet. Test carefully. Human Food Bar's website mentions *"the benefits of olive oil greatly depending on how the olives are sourced and oil is made"*. For example, vacuum-extracted olive oil is thought to be better as the process reduces exposure to oxygen and keeps polyphenols (anti-oxidants) (source: *Apollo Olive Oil*). As extra-virgin olive oil is the least processed form of olive oil, opt for vacuum-extracted extra-virgin olive oil.

Oxalates: The site VP Foundation notes this is low oxalate, and we consider it an excellent healthy choice.

Salicylates: Olive oil is made from olives which can be high in salicylates depending on the type. Olive oil is similarly thought to be in the highish range of salicylate content.

Olives

- DASH: Fat: ✘ Sodium: ✘ Sugar: ✔
- Diverticulitis: Stage 1: ✘ Stage 2: ✔ Stage 3: ✘
- Histamine: ✘
- Lectin: ✔
- Oxalate: ✘
- Salicylates: ✘

DASH Diet (Hypertension): Olives are high in saturated fat and sodium. Limit or avoid on the DASH diet. *Saturated fat content: 1.2g (per 100g), Sodium content: 880 mg (per 100g), 38% daily value based on a 2,000 calorie diet, Sugar content: 0g (per 100g)* (source: *Fatsecret Platform API*).

Diverticulitis: No solid foods can be eaten at stage one, the clear liquids diet. Low in fiber, so allowed on the low-fiber diet.

Histamine: As good as olive oil is, frustratingly, olives aren't as good on our list.

Lectins: As per olive oil, olives contain some lectins, but as they're full of antioxidants and healthy monounsaturated fats, the benefits outweigh the negatives. It's thought that they can be eaten without restriction, and it's unnecessary to eliminate them from your diet. Test carefully.

Oxalates: The University of Chicago classifies them as very high with 18mg per 100 g. Best to avoid.

Salicylates: While some reliable sources list olives as potentially high in salicylates, black olives are lower, coming in at .34 mg per 100 g. Green olives tend to test much higher at over 1 mg per 100 g.

Onion

- DASH: Fat: ✔ Sodium: ✔ Sugar: ✔
- Diverticulitis: Stage 1: ✘ Stage 2: ✘ Stage 3: ✔
- Histamine: 🤔
- Lectin: ✔
- Oxalate: ✔
- Salicylates: 🤔

DASH Diet (Hypertension): Allowed. Onions are a great way to enhance flavor without adding extra salt to a meal. *Saturated fat content: 0g (per 100g), Sodium content: 4mg (per 100g), less than 1% daily value based on a 2,000 calorie diet, Sugar content: 4.2g (per 100g).*

Diverticulitis: No solid foods can be eaten at stage one, the clear liquids diet. Allowed on the high-fiber diet.

Histamine: Test carefully.

Lectins: Onions fall under the lowest lectin content options for a low lectin diet.

Oxalates: Low oxalate.

Salicylates: There is plenty of debate about onions and salicylates. Most sources seem to agree that the levels of salicylates are not extremely high, but they still need to be approached with caution. Fresh onions, according to multiple trustworthy analyses, including a study published in the Journal of the American Dietetic Association Vol. 85:8 1985, have been found to contain .16 mg to .18 mg of salicylates per 100 g, placing them in the "low level" category. However, other food lists and studies believe salicylate levels in onions are higher. Onions are rich in powerful antioxidants, and other compounds are known to fight inflammation and reduce triglycerides and cholesterol levels which can lower heart disease risk. Hence, they are something that you may want to retain on your low salicylate diet.

Orange

- DASH: Fat: ✓ Sodium: ✓ Sugar: ✗
- Diverticulitis: Stage 1: ✓ Stage 2: ✗ Stage 3: ✓
- Histamine: ✗
- Lectin: 😬
- Oxalate: ✗
- Salicylates: ✗

DASH Diet (Hypertension): Oranges are high in sugar but can be included in moderation on the DASH diet. *Saturated fat content: 0g (per 100g), Sodium content: 0g (per 100g), 0% daily value based on a 2,000 calorie diet, Sugar content: 9g (per 100g).*

Diverticulitis: Allowed on the high-fiber diet.

Histamine: Most citrus seems to be very high in histamine.

Lectins: Opinion is split. One source confirmed oranges are a source of lectins. However, another source noted oranges contain D-Mannose, a powerful natural lectin-blocker. Test carefully.

Oxalates: Generally high and best avoided. Peel especially so. Oxalate content may depend on the size. A small orange (2⅜" diameter) is classified as moderate with 10–25 mg oxalates. One teaspoon of raw orange peel contains 10–25 mg of oxalates. Orange juice is high in oxalates (source: *St. Joseph's Healthcare Hamilton*).

Salicylates: Oranges are thought to contain a high level of salicylates

Oregano

- DASH: Fat: ✗ Sodium: ✓ Sugar: ✓
- Diverticulitis: Stage 1: 😬 Stage 2: ✓ Stage 3: ✗
- Histamine: ✓
- Lectin: ✗
- Oxalate: 😬
- Salicylates: ✗

DASH Diet (Hypertension): Oregano can be used in moderation to add flavor to dishes. *Saturated fat content: 2.66g (per 100g), Sodium content: 15mg (per 100g), 1% daily value based on a 2,000 calorie diet, Sugar content: 4g (per 100g).*

Diverticulitis: Low in fiber, so allowed on the low-fiber diet.

Histamine: Both fresh and dried seem to be tolerated well.

Lectins: Contains some lectins. Depends on the quantities used. Dr Suzanne Joy S Stuart of Naturally Balanced Health recommends limiting or avoiding oregano.

Oxalates: Low to moderate, dried oregano is listed as having 5 - 10 mg per 100 grams (source: *Urinary Stones - Low Oxalate List*).

Salicylates: Spices tend to be high in salicylates. Oregano is another spice that is high in salicylates.

Ostrich

- DASH: Fat: ✓ Sodium: ✓ Sugar: ✓
- Diverticulitis: Stage 1: ✗ Stage 2: ✓ Stage 3: ✗
- Histamine: ✓
- Lectin: ✓
- Oxalate: ✓
- Salicylates: ✓

Not admittedly, a common food, but it still makes it into our food list.

DASH Diet (Hypertension): Allowed. Ostrich is a meat option that is low in sodium and saturated fat. *Saturated fat content: 1g (per 100g), Sodium content: 80mg (per 100g), 3% daily value based on a 2,000 calorie diet, Sugar content: 0g (per 100g).*

Diverticulitis: No solid foods can be eaten at stage one, the clear liquids diet. Meat contains no fiber, so ostrich is allowed on the low-fiber diet.

Histamine: Note other comments about fresh meat elsewhere. No leftovers.

Lectins: Fine on a low-lectin diet. Opt for pasture-raised meat when possible.

Oxalates: Low oxalate. However, eating large portions of meat can potentially increase the risk of kidney stones.

Salicylates: Despite coming from a bird, ostrich tastes more like premium beef and is rich in iron while lower in fat and cholesterol and free from salicylates. For more information, see "Meat"

Oyster

- DASH: Fat: ✗ Sodium: ✗ Sugar: ✓
- Diverticulitis: Stage 1: ✗ Stage 2: ✓ Stage 3: ✗
- Histamine: ✗
- Lectin: ✓
- Oxalate: ✓
- Salicylates: ✓

DASH Diet (Hypertension): Oysters are high in saturated fat and sodium. Try to limit or avoid on the DASH diet. *Saturated fat content: 3.2g (per 100g), Sodium content: 417mg (per 100g), 17% daily value based on a 2,000 calorie diet, Sugar content: 0g (per 100g).*

Diverticulitis: No solid foods can be eaten at stage one, the clear liquids diet. Seafood contains no fiber, so oyster is allowed on the low-fiber diet.

Histamine: Avoid.

Lectins: Full of health benefits. Oysters are high in protein, vitamin D, zinc, iron and copper (source: *Gourmet Food Store*), plus they're permitted on a low-lectin diet.

Oxalates: Low, less than 5 mg per 100 grams (source: *https://www.urinarystones.info/resources/Docs/Oxalate-content-of-food-2008.pdf*)

Salicylates: See "Bivalves"

Papaya

- DASH: Fat: ✓ Sodium: ✓ Sugar: ✗
- Diverticulitis: Stage 1: ✗ Stage 2: 😐 Stage 3: ✓
- Histamine: ✗
- Lectin: ✓
- Oxalate: ✓
- Salicylates: ✓

DASH Diet (Hypertension): Papayas are high in lycopene and Vitamin C, which may help prevent heart disease. Include in moderation as part of a healthy diet. *Saturated fat content: 0.04g (per 100g), Sodium content: 3mg (per 100g), less than 1% daily value based on a 2,000 calorie diet, Sugar content: 5.9g (per 100g)* (source: *Fatsecret Platform API*).

Diverticulitis: No solid foods can be eaten at stage one, the clear liquids diet. Ripe papaya is allowed on a low-fiber diet.

Histamine: One of the fruits most likely to cause a reaction.

Lectins: Acceptable.

Oxalates: Contains little to no oxalates.

Salicylates: Papaya is one of the lowest salicylate fruits. We even considered putting papaya on the cover of this food dictionary. It is low in salicylates and loaded with nutrients. It's particularly rich in vitamins A, C, and antioxidants to help reduce the risk of cancer.

Parsley

- DASH: Fat: ✓ Sodium: ✓ Sugar: ✓
- Diverticulitis: Stage 1: 😐 Stage 2: ✓ Stage 3: ✗
- Histamine: ✓
- Lectin: ✗
- Oxalate: 😐
- Salicylates: 😐

Parsley is full of health-boosting vitamins such as vitamins A, C, and K (source: *Real Simple*).

DASH Diet (Hypertension): Allowed. *Saturated fat content: 0.1g (per 100g), Sodium content: 56mg (per 100g) 2% daily value based on a 2,000 calorie diet, Sugar content: 0.9g (per 100g).*

Diverticulitis: Low in fiber, so allowed on the low-fiber diet.

Histamine: Acceptable.

Lectins: Contains some lectins.

Oxalates: Plenty of debate. Fresh parsley contains 5–10 mg per 100 grams, making it low to moderate in oxalates (source: *https://www.urinarystones.info/resources/Docs/Oxalate-content-of-food-2008.pdf*). Others disagree. The Agriculture Handbook No. 8-11, Vegetables and Vegetable Products, 1984, lists Parsley as very high in oxalates. The Heal With Food website notes parsley and chives; *Like parsley, chives are only used in small amounts in cooking. Therefore, chives are not likely to contribute much oxalic acid to your diet, although they are among the most concentrated dietary sources of oxalates. A 100-serving of chives is estimated to provide 1480 milligrams of oxalates.*

Salicylates: This is one where emerging research is changing the way we think about an ingredient. Parsley was initially believed to be low in salicylates, but reliable sources have noted recent research revealing the opposite to be true. This has led to a lot of conflicting information, with it ranked as low, moderate, or high. Frustrating, we know, but that's why this food list is important as if you relied on one list, you wouldn't know this. Consider this when making your decision whether to include it in your diet. Eat small amounts before you know how your body will react.

Parsnip

- DASH: Fat: ✓ Sodium: ✓ Sugar: ✓
- Diverticulitis: Stage 1: ✗ Stage 2: ✗ Stage 3: ✓
- Histamine: ✓
- Lectin: ✓
- Oxalate: ✗
- Salicylates: 😐

Parsnips are rich in fiber and antioxidants (source: *BBC Good Food*).

DASH Diet (Hypertension): Allowed. *Saturated fat content: 0.1g (per 100g), Sodium content: 10mg (per 100g) less than 1% daily value based on a 2,000 calorie diet, Sugar content: 4.8g (per 100g).*

Diverticulitis: No solid foods can be eaten at stage one, the clear liquids diet. Allowed on the high-fiber diet.

Histamine: We love the humble parsnip. Be warned, it can go off quickly though, so eat fresh.

Lectins: Acceptable. This is an effective alternative to potato, which is high in lectins. One to put on your 'avoid' list.

Oxalates: High in oxalates, 15 mg per 100 g (*University of Chicago*).

Salicylates: Parsnip contains a moderate amount of salicylates.

Passionfruit

- DASH: Fat: ✓ Sodium: ✓ Sugar: ✗
- Diverticulitis: Stage 1: ✗ Stage 2: ✗ Stage 3: ✓
- Histamine: ✓
- Lectin: ✓
- Oxalate: ✓
- Salicylates: ✗

DASH Diet (Hypertension): Passionfruit is high in sugar. Try to limit or avoid on the DASH diet. *Saturated fat content: 0.1g (per 100g), Sodium content: 28mg (per 100g), 1% daily value based on a 2,000 calorie diet, Sugar content: 11g (per 100g).*

Diverticulitis: No solid foods can be eaten at stage one, the clear liquids diet. Acceptable on the high-fiber diet.

Histamine: Allowed.

Lectins: Allowed. Consume when passion fruit is in-season.

Oxalates: Low.

Salicylates: While passion fruit is often rated as high in salicylates, some food lists demur and say it is lower. Most fruits contain a high amount, so we've decided to err on the side of caution.

Pasta

- DASH: Fat: ✓ Sodium: ✓ Sugar: ✓
- Diverticulitis: Stage 1: ✗ Stage 2: ✓ Stage 3: ✓
- Histamine: 🤐
- Lectin: 🤐
- Oxalate: ✗
- Salicylates: 🤐

DASH Diet (Hypertension): Allowed. Choose whole grain options when eating pasta. *Saturated fat content: 0.2g (per 100g), Sodium content: 6mg (per 100g), less than 1% daily value based on a 2,000 calorie diet, Sugar content: 0.6g (per 100g).*

Diverticulitis: No solid foods can be eaten at stage one, the clear liquids diet. White pasta is low in fiber. Go for whole-grain pasta if you're on a high-fiber diet.

Histamine: Depends on the ingredients used, for example, corn pasta is acceptable but test wheat pasta carefully. Pea Pasta may cause issues, and chickpea flour is used in some gluten-free pasta which is a no-no.

Lectins: It depends on what the pasta is made from. Wheat flour contains a lectin called wheat germ agglutinin (WGA). A study found variable amounts of WGA in wholemeal pasta *"probably as a consequence of thermal inactivation during food processing"* (source: *Temperature-dependent decay of wheat germ agglutinin activity and its implications for food processing and analysis*). It seems that cooking reduces lectin content. Opt for whole-wheat pasta. Another study found: *"Commercial pasta products labeled as whole wheat were also tested for WGA content and found to contain up to 90% less WGA compared to a whole grain standard."* (source: *Killilea DW, McQueen R, Abegania JR. Wheat germ agglutinin is a biomarker of whole grain content in wheat flour and pasta*). There is also an array of non-wheat pasta available, and you can check the individual ingredients on this list. For example, there is pasta on sale made from almond flour (with skin removed) which may be a better choice on a low-lectin diet.

Oxalates: High in oxalates. Most pasta contains 20-30 mg per 100g (source: *Science Direct*). You could try pasta alternatives that are lower oxalate (check individual ingredients in this guide).

Salicylates: Depends on the ingredients used, for example, pasta made from corn or maize starch is allowed as the salicylates have been removed during processing. Avoid pasta made from corn or maize flour as this is high in salicylates.

Peach

- DASH: Fat: ✓ Sodium: ✓ Sugar: ✗
- Diverticulitis: Stage 1: ✗ Stage 2: 🤐 Stage 3: ✓
- Histamine: ✓
- Lectin: ✓
- Oxalate: ✓
- Salicylates: ✗

DASH Diet (Hypertension): Some studies have shown that peaches contain compounds that may reduce the risk of heart disease (source: *Healthline*). Eat in moderation. *Saturated fat content: 0.01g (per 100g), Sodium content: 0mg (per 100g), less than 1% daily value based on a 2,000 calorie diet, Sugar content: 8.4g (per 100g)* (source: *Fatsecret Platform API*).

Diverticulitis: No solid foods can be eaten at stage one, the clear liquids diet. Ripe peach with no skin is allowed on the low-fiber diet.

Histamine: We like to buy, chop and freeze and use in small portions in desserts.

Lectins: Allowed. As with most fruit on our food list, ideally eat when peaches are in season, although this may not always be possible, peaches should still be fine.

Oxalates: Thought to be low in oxalate and a good choice, although some disparity between lists.

Salicylates: Both fresh and canned peaches contain a moderately high amount of salicylates.

Peanuts

- DASH: Fat: ✗ Sodium: ✓ Sugar: ✓
- Diverticulitis: Stage 1: ✗ Stage 2: ✗ Stage 3: ✓
- Histamine: ✗
- Lectin: ✗
- Oxalate: ✗
- Salicylates: ✗

DASH Diet (Hypertension): Although nuts such as peanuts contain little sodium naturally, they're often sold covered in salt. Make sure to choose no sodium or low sodium when purchasing them. *Saturated fat content: 7g (per 100g), Sodium content: 18mg (per 100g) less than 1% daily value based on a 2,000 calorie diet, Sugar content: 4g (per 100g).*

Diverticulitis: No solid foods can be eaten at stage one, the clear liquids diet. Allowed on the high-fiber diet.

Histamine: One of the worst nuts for histamine.

Lectins: High in lectins. It's thought that cooking peanuts may not eliminate their lectin content. Avoid peanuts and also peanut butter.

Oxalates: Thought to be very high in oxalates, like many nuts.

Salicylates: Peanuts are thought to be very high in salicylates. One to avoid on a low salicylate diet. Web MD notes; *"Cereals that contain almonds or peanuts are high in salicylates and should be avoided"*. The website drugs.com also notes peanuts are high in salicylates. Naturally Savvy notes the following food products may also contain salicylates; *"Nuts such as pine nuts, peanuts, pistachios, and almonds"*.

Pear

- DASH: Fat: ✓ Sodium: ✓ Sugar: ✗
- Diverticulitis: Stage 1: ✗ Stage 2: ✗ Stage 3: ✓
- Histamine: 😷
- Lectin: ✓
- Oxalate: ✓
- Salicylates: ✓

DASH Diet (Hypertension): Pears are high in sugar but rich in flavonoids that promote heart health and low blood pressure (source: *BBC Good Food*). Eat in moderation. *Saturated fat content: 0g (per 100g), Sodium content: 1mg (per 100g), less than 1% daily value based on a 2,000 calorie diet, Sugar content: 10g (per 100g).*

Diverticulitis: No solid foods can be eaten at stage one, the clear liquids diet. Allowed on the high-fiber diet.

Histamine: If canned, then likely to be higher in histamine than fresh.

Lectins: Acceptable.

Oxalates: Low.

Salicylates: Pears are another fruit we considered putting on the front cover of this food dictionary. They can be very low in salicylates but only under certain conditions. Peeling your pear is key. If you peel a pear before eating it, it will have no salicylates or only a trace amount; however, unpeeled pears may be quite high in salicylates.

Peas (green)

- DASH: Fat: ✓ Sodium: ✓ Sugar: ✗
- Diverticulitis: Stage 1: ✗ Stage 2: ✗ Stage 3: ✓
- Histamine: 😖
- Lectin: 😖
- Oxalate: ✓
- Salicylates: ✓

Peas contain omega-3 and omega-6 fatty acids that reduce oxidation and inflammation in the body (source: *WebMD*).

DASH Diet (Hypertension): Watch the sugar content. *Saturated fat content: 0.1g (per 100g), Sodium content: 5 mg (per 100g), less than 1% daily value based on a 2,000 calorie diet, Sugar content: 6g (per 100g).*

Diverticulitis: No solid foods can be eaten at stage one, the clear liquids diet. Allowed on the high-fiber diet.

Histamine: Peas are a weird one. We do well with them, however having canvassed the histamine community, many people do struggle with them. Mast Cell 360 lists green split peas and yellow split peas as low histamine, just "peas" as high histamine.

Lectins: Mixed opinion. Some say they contain low levels of lectins and are safe to eat. However, others believe they may interfere with gut absorption. A study found that soaking peas *"significantly decreased the contents of lectins"* (source: *Shi L, Arntfield SD, Nickerson M. Changes in levels of phytic acid, lectins and oxalates during soaking and cooking of Canadian pulses*). Limit consumption and test carefully initially.

Oxalates: Boiled peas are thought to be very low in oxalate.

Salicylates: Fresh green peas may have a low amount of salicylates, up to .25 mg per 100 g.

Pea Shoots (or pea sprouts)

- DASH: Fat: ✓ Sodium: ✓ Sugar: ✓
- Diverticulitis: Stage 1: ✗ Stage 2: ✗ Stage 3: ✓
- Histamine: ✓
- Lectin: ✗
- Oxalate: 😖
- Salicylates: ✗

There is a slight difference here. Pea sprouts are seeds grown in a jar (without soil), whereas pea shoots are plants grown in the soil.

DASH Diet (Hypertension): Allowed. They're also a great source of fiber, vitamins A, C, and K and potassium (source: *Science Direct*). *Saturated fat content: 0g, Sodium content: 0mg, Sugar content: 3g (per 70g)* (source: *Fatsecret Platform API*).

Diverticulitis: No solid foods can be eaten at stage one, the clear liquids diet. Allowed on the high-fiber diet.

Histamine: Believed to be histamine-lowering. A superb addition to your shopping list.

Lectins: Seeds are high in lectins, so we suggest limiting the consumption of pea sprouts. Test pea shoots carefully as these are a part of the pea family.

Oxalates: Difficult to find consistent data, but eating moderate amounts of microgreens is less likely to cause the formation of kidney stones because of the higher citrate levels in micro greens which counterbalance the formation of calcium oxalate. Test carefully.

Salicylates: The latest food chemical chart from Royal Prince Alfred Hospital's Allergy Unit (RPAH), the world's leading allergy unit in terms of food chemicals like salicylates, notes that they contain a high amount. This is a shame because they can be very healthy in other aspects and even histamine-lowering too, but proceed with great caution. There isn't, however, a lot of information on pea shoots in relation to salicylates, so we await further research.

Peppermint tea
- DASH: Fat: ✓ Sodium: ✓ Sugar: ✓
- Diverticulitis: Stage 1: ✓ Stage 2: ✓ Stage 3: ✗
- Histamine: ✓
- Lectin: ✓
- Oxalate: ✓
- Salicylates: ✗

DASH Diet (Hypertension): Allowed. Choose teas such as peppermint tea as a healthier alternative to sugary drinks. *Saturated fat content: 0g (per 100g), Sodium content: 0mg (per 100g) 0% daily value based on a 2,000 calorie diet, Sugar content: 0g (per 100g).*

Diverticulitis: Tea with no milk or cream is allowed at stage one, the clear liquid diet. Also allowed on the low-fiber diet.

Histamine: Acceptable.

Lectins: It's thought that tea is permitted on a low-lectin diet.

Oxalates: Low; just 0.41 mg per cup (source: *Pubmed, National Library of Medicine*).

Salicylates: As a herbal tea, peppermint also contains a high level of salicylates.

Pickled food
- DASH: Fat: ✓ Sodium: ✗ Sugar: ✓
- Diverticulitis: Stage 1: ✗ Stage 2: ✗ Stage 3: ✓
- Histamine: ✗
- Lectin: ✓
- Oxalate: ✗
- Salicylates: ✗

DASH Diet (Hypertension): Pickled foods are thought to be very high in sodium because of the brining process. Go for low-sodium options and eat in moderation. *Saturated fat content: 0.082g (per 100g), Sodium content: 1,061mg (per 100g), Sugar content: 2.74g (per 100g) (source: Fatsecret Platform API).*

Diverticulitis: No solid foods can be eaten at stage one, the clear liquids diet. Allowed on the high-fiber diet.

Histamine: All pickled food should be avoided. Watch out for pickled gherkins in burgers!

Lectins: Acceptable.

Oxalates: Dill pickles are very low, and pickled beets are extremely high.

Salicylates: Royal Prince Alfred Hospital's Allergy Unit (RPAH), the world's leading allergy unit in terms of food chemicals like salicylates, (mentioned above), lists all pickled foods, including pickles, pickled cucumber, pickled olives, and pickled onions as very high in salicylates.

Pineapple

- DASH: Fat: ✓ Sodium: ✓ Sugar: ✗
- Diverticulitis: Stage 1: ✗ Stage 2: ✗ Stage 3: ✓
- Histamine: ✗
- Lectin: ✓
- Oxalate: ✗
- Salicylates: ✗

DASH Diet (Hypertension): If you're buying canned fruits like pineapple, make sure you buy them canned in their own juice and not syrup to avoid extra sugar. Pineapple is high in sugar but can be consumed occasionally in the DASH diet. *Saturated fat content: 0g (per 100g), Sodium content: 1mg (per 100g), less than 1% daily value based on a 2,000 calorie diet, Sugar content: 10g (per 100g).*

Diverticulitis: No solid foods can be eaten at stage one, the clear liquids diet. Allowed on the high-fiber diet.

Histamine: On the Healing Histamine Site, author Yasmina got to where she could eat high histamine foods whenever she wanted, though she always chose high nutrient, healing foods, and didn't eat them at every meal. She notes how important it is to reintroduce 'healthy' higher histamine foods such as pineapple once you start to feel better, and we wholeheartedly agree.

Lectins: Acceptable however, note the high sugar content.

Oxalates: Low if fresh. Dried pineapple is very high, with half a cup containing 30 mg (source: *St. Joseph's Healthcare Hamilton*). Canned pineapple is also to be avoided.

Salicylates: Very high in salicylates.

Pistachio

- DASH: Fat: ✗ Sodium: ✓ Sugar: ✗
- Diverticulitis: Stage 1: ✗ Stage 2: ✗ Stage 3: ✓
- Histamine: 🤔
- Lectin: 🤔
- Oxalate: ✗
- Salicylates: ✗

Pistachios are a heart-healthy nut option.

DASH Diet (Hypertension): Eat in moderation as they're high in saturated fat and sugar. *Saturated fat content: 6g (per 100g), Sodium content: 1mg (per 100g) less than 1% daily value based on a 2,000 calorie diet, Sugar content: 8g (per 100g).*

Diverticulitis: No solid foods can be eaten at stage one, the clear liquids diet. Allowed on the high-fiber diet.

Histamine: Test carefully.

Lectins: This is a nut where opinion is mixed, and one reason we wrote this book is that major lists often disagree. For example, it's thought to be low lectin according to the website Healthline, but multiple other research sources show pistachios as containing problematic lectins. Test carefully, and we will update this list as new research becomes available.

Oxalates: 14 mg per 1/4 cup (source: *https://www.thekidneydietitian.org/low-oxalate-nuts/#Pistachios*). And who only eats 1/4 cup of pistachios at once? 49 mg per 100g (source: *PainSpy Low Oxalate Diet Foods List*).

Salicylates: Pistachio nuts contain quite a high amount of salicylates - often over .5 mg per 100 g. Healthline says they are rich in healthy fats, antioxidants, protein, and various nutrients like vitamin B6. Unless you're very sensitive, you may consume a very limited amount (one to three pistachios) without negative effects. But one to three pistachios doesn't sound much fun - sorry!

Plum

- DASH: Fat: ✓ Sodium: ✓ Sugar: ✗
- Diverticulitis: Stage 1: ✗ Stage 2: 😐 Stage 3: ✓
- Histamine: 😐
- Lectin: ✓
- Oxalate: ✓
- Salicylates: 😐

DASH Diet (Hypertension): The potassium in plums is good for lowering blood pressure (source: *WebMD*). Include in moderation as a healthy part of the DASH diet. *Saturated fat content: 0g (per 100g), Sodium content: 0mg (per 100g), less than 1% daily value based on a 2,000 calorie diet, Sugar content: 10g (per 100g).*

Diverticulitis: No solid foods can be eaten at stage one, the clear liquids diet. Allowed on the low-fiber diet if ripe and no skin.

Histamine: Test carefully.

Lectins: Low in lectins.

Oxalates: Thought to contain little to no oxalates.

Salicylates: Plums are difficult to rate. We advise you to avoid canned plums and if you decide to eat fresh plums, start with a small amount until you know how your body will react. Fresh plums are thought to be lower in salicylates than canned plums, but the salicylate community is divided on whether plums are low or high in salicylates.

Pomegranate

- DASH: Fat: ✓ Sodium: ✓ Sugar: ✗
- Diverticulitis: Stage 1: ✗ Stage 2: ✗ Stage 3: ✓
- Histamine: ✓
- Lectin: ✓
- Oxalate: ✗
- Salicylates: ✗

Loaded with vitamin C.

DASH Diet (Hypertension): Pomegranate is high in sugar. Try to eat in moderation. *Saturated fat content: 0.1g (per 100g), Sodium content: 3mg (per 100g), less 1% daily value based on a 2,000 calorie diet, Sugar content: 14g (per 100g).*

Diverticulitis: No solid foods can be eaten at stage one, the clear liquids diet. Allowed on the high-fiber diet.

Histamine: Thought by many to be histamine lowering, so an excellent option for you. Pomegranate seeds are delicious in salads.

Lectins: Tolerated.

Oxalates: High.

Salicylates: Unfortunately, after extensive research, we found most trustworthy sites categorize pomegranates as high in salicylates. An analysis by the ADA found pomegranates to be very low in salicylates. Who's right then? Unfortunately, as always, this is an area where you will have to work out your own tolerance level to pomegranate.

Poppy seeds
- DASH: Fat: ✗ Sodium: ✓ Sugar: ✓
- Diverticulitis: Stage 1: ✗ Stage 2: ✗ Stage 3: ✓
- Histamine: 😐
- Lectin: ✗
- Oxalate: ✗
- Salicylates: ✓

DASH Diet (Hypertension): Poppy seeds are high in saturated fat. Try to limit or avoid. *Saturated fat content: 4.5 g (per 100g), Sodium content: 26mg (per 100g), 1% daily value based on a 2,000 calorie diet, Sugar content: 3g (per 100g).*

Diverticulitis: No solid foods can be eaten at stage one, the clear liquids diet. Allowed on the high-fiber diet.

Histamine: Test carefully.

Lectins: High in lectins. One to put on your 'avoid' list.

Oxalates: High.

Salicylates: Negligible amount of salicylates.

Pork
- DASH: Fat: ✗ Sodium: ✓ Sugar: ✓
- Diverticulitis: Stage 1: ✗ Stage 2: ✓ Stage 3: ✗
- Histamine: ✓
- Lectin: ✓
- Oxalate: ✗
- Salicylates: ✓

DASH Diet (Hypertension): Pork is high in saturated fat. To limit fat intake, choose leaner proteins like poultry on the DASH diet. *Saturated fat content: 5g (per 100g), Sodium content: 62mg (per 100g) 2% daily value based on a 2,000 calorie diet, Sugar content: 0g (per 100g).*

Diverticulitis: No solid foods can be eaten at stage one, the clear liquids diet. Meat contains no fiber, so pork is allowed on the low-fiber diet.

Histamine: As long as organic and freshly cooked - pork is acceptable. Non-organic would be a poorer choice. No leftovers.

Lectins: Tolerated. Opt for grass-fed meat for a much healthier dish.

Oxalates: High.

Salicylates: See "Meat"

Potato
- DASH: Fat: ✓ Sodium: ✓ Sugar: ✓
- Diverticulitis: Stage 1: ✗ Stage 2: ✓ Stage 3: ✓

- Histamine: ✓
- Lectin: ✗
- Oxalate: ✗
- Salicylates: 😬

DASH Diet (Hypertension): Potatoes are high in potassium, making them a good inclusion in the DASH diet (source: *CBS News*). Eat in moderation to limit sodium intake. *Saturated fat content: 0.5g (per 100g), Sodium content: 254mg (per 100g), 11% daily value based on a 2,000 calorie diet, Sugar content: 0.8g (per 100g).*

Diverticulitis: No solid foods can be eaten at stage one, the clear liquids diet. Remember to peel the potatoes on a low-fiber diet. Potatoes may be eaten with their skin on a high-fiber diet.

Histamine: Low histamine and applies to all potato types. Includes sweet potatoes too.

Lectins: Potatoes are high in lectins. Although cooking reduces lectin content, it's thought that potato lectins are quite resistant and will only reduce by 50-60% (source: *The Woodlands Institute for health and wellness*).

Oxalates: Dr. Jockers lists potatoes in his High-Oxalate Foods list. A medium baked potato has 50 mg of oxalates per 100g according to the Pain Spy Low Oxalate Foods List, but other sources say you can lower this by getting rid of the skin. (This is also considered to be the same with pears which are lower oxalate when you take the skin off). That's where many of the oxalates are. The skin contains fiber, vitamin C, B vitamins, and other healthy nutrients (source: *St. Joseph's Healthcare Hamilton*).

Salicylates: The next time you make mashed potatoes, use your peeler to avoid salicylates. Peeled white potatoes are thought to be free of salicylates, while unpeeled white potatoes contain a low amount, up to .25 mg per 100 g. So potatoes are a bit like pears. Potato and pear salad, anyone? Ignore us, let's continue. Be aware that not all potatoes are created equal. Red potatoes and yellow sweet potatoes have a moderate amount of salicylates, and sweet potatoes are considered high in salicylates and oxalates. In summary, if you're not ultra-sensitive to salicylates but want to maximize nutrition choose unpeeled white potatoes. The skin offers a good amount of fiber, B vitamins, vitamin C, and other beneficial nutrients. If you are ultra-sensitive - peel 'em.

Poultry meat

- DASH: Fat: ✗ Sodium: ✓ Sugar: ✓
- Diverticulitis: Stage 1: ✗ Stage 2: ✓ Stage 3: ✗
- Histamine: ✓
- Lectin: ✓
- Oxalate: ✓
- Salicylates: ✗

DASH Diet (Hypertension): Choose lean poultry meats like turkey and chicken on the DASH diet. *Saturated fat content: 7g (per 100g), Sodium content: 40mg (per 100g), 1% daily value based on a 2,000 calorie diet, Sugar content: 0g (per 100g).*

Diverticulitis: No solid foods can be eaten at stage one, the clear liquids diet. Meat contains no fiber, so it is allowed on a low-fiber diet.

Histamine: As long as it is organic and very fresh. Non-organic would be a poorer choice. No leftovers.

Lectins: Tolerated. Opt for pastured poultry meat.

Oxalates: Low oxalate. However, eating large portions of meat can potentially increase the risk of kidney stones. Non-organic would also potentially be a poorer choice on the general health front.

Salicylates: See "Meat"

Prawn

- DASH: Fat: ✓ Sodium: ✓ Sugar: ✓
- Diverticulitis: Stage 1: ✗ Stage 2: ✓ Stage 3: ✗
- Histamine: ✗
- Lectin: ✗
- Oxalate: ✓
- Salicylates: ✗

DASH Diet (Hypertension): Allowed. Prawns can be a great source of protein.

Diverticulitis: No solid foods can be eaten at stage one, the clear liquids diet. Seafood contains no fiber, so prawns are allowed on the low-fiber diet.

Histamine: Avoid.

Lectins: Closely related to shrimp, many believe these could also be a source of lectins.

Oxalates: Low, like most seafood.

Salicylates: See "Fish" while keeping in mind that fried versions may contain salicylates and other ingredients that do not support optimal health. Prawns are the one fish noted by the Food Can Make You Ill website to avoid.

Processed cheese

- DASH: Fat: ✗ Sodium: ✗ Sugar: ✗
- Diverticulitis: Stage 1: ✗ Stage 2: ✓ Stage 3: ✗
- Histamine: ✗
- Lectin: ✗
- Oxalate: ✓
- Salicylates: ✓

Processed cheese is mixed with artificial ingredients such as flavor enhancers, coloring etc. it can no longer be classified as cheese.

DASH Diet (Hypertension): Try to limit or avoid intake of processed cheese on the DASH diet. *Saturated fat content: 6g (per 100g), Sodium content: 1,705mg (per 100g), 71% daily value based on a 2,000 calorie diet, Sugar content: 8g (per 100g).*

Diverticulitis: No solid foods can be eaten at stage one, the clear liquids diet. Cheese contains no fiber, so they're allowed on a low-fiber diet.

Histamine: The words processed and cheese both = high histamine.

Lectins: These contain 2-3 times more sodium than unprocessed cheese (source: *Ricardo Cuisine*). The lectin content depends on the type of cheese used in the process, but given that these aren't as healthy as regular cheese, we recommend limiting processed cheese consumption. If eating processed cheese, opt for cheese produced from A2 milk (from cows originating in the Channel Islands and Southern France). Easier said than done, we know. Knowing the type of milk used during cheese production will help you assess. Test carefully.

Oxalates: See cheese.

Salicylates: Most cheeses are thought to be very low in salicylates. But keep in mind that processed cheese is high in sodium and saturated fat along with unhealthy additives. Regular consumption can lead to obesity and hypertension, the reason for our ranking.

Prune

- DASH: Fat: ✔ Sodium: ✔ Sugar: ✗
- Diverticulitis: Stage 1: ✗ Stage 2: ✗ Stage 3: ✔
- Histamine: 😬
- Lectin: ✔
- Oxalate: ✗
- Salicylates: ✗

A dried plum.

DASH Diet (Hypertension): High in sugar. Try to limit or avoid. *Saturated fat content: 0.1g (per 100g), Sodium content: 2 mg (per 100g) less than 1% daily value based on a 2,000 calorie diet, Sugar content: 38g (per 100g).*

Diverticulitis: No solid foods can be eaten at stage one, the clear liquids diet. Allowed on the high-fiber diet.

Histamine: Test carefully.

Lectins: As plums are low in lectin content, permitted.

Oxalates: Dried prune is very high in oxalates. Prune juice is thought to be moderate in oxalates. Proceed with caution.

Salicylates: Thought to be extremely high in salicylates. Indeed, there are possibly more salicylates in prunes than in any other fruit. The website Allergenics notes; *"Dried fruits such as apricots, raisins, dates and prunes have extremely high levels."*

Pulses

- DASH: Fat: ✔ Sodium: ✔ Sugar: ✗
- Diverticulitis: Stage 1: ✗ Stage 2: ✗ Stage 3: ✔
- Histamine: ✗
- Lectin: ✗
- Oxalate: ✗
- Salicylates: Check the individual pulse for details.

Pulses include peas, lentils, fava beans, chickpeas, and common beans.

DASH Diet (Hypertension): High in sugar, so try to eat in moderation. *Saturated fat content: 0.1g (per 100g), Sodium content: 5 mg (per 100g) less than 1% daily value based on a 2,000 calorie diet, Sugar content: 6g (per 100g).*

Diverticulitis: No solid foods can be eaten at stage one, the clear liquids diet. Allowed on the high-fiber diet.

Histamine: See "beans" for more info.

Lectins: Beans, peas, and lentils are all high in lectins to varying degrees. Check individual ingredients.

Oxalates: Check individual ingredients. According to PubMed, pulses can be very high in oxalates. Oxalate content varies, ranging from 244.7-294.0 mg/100 g in peas, 168.6-289.1 mg/100 g in lentils, 241.5-291.4 mg/100 g in fava beans, 92.2-214.0 mg/100 g in chickpeas and 98.86-117.0 mg/100 g in common beans. Approximately 24-72% of total oxalate appeared to be soluble in all investigated pulses. It notes; *Soaking the seeds in distilled water significantly decreased the contents of total oxalate (17.40-51.89%) and soluble oxalate (26.66-56.29%).*

Salicylates: Pulses include common beans, peas, chickpeas, fava beans, and lentils, all of which vary in salicylates, from a low amount in chickpeas to a high level in fava beans. Check the individual pulse for details.

Pumpkin seed oil

- DASH: Fat: ✗ Sodium: ✓ Sugar: ✓
- Diverticulitis: Stage 1: ✗ Stage 2: ✗ Stage 3: ✓
- Histamine: ✓
- Lectin: ✗
- Oxalate: 😐
- Salicylates: 😐

DASH Diet (Hypertension): High in polyunsaturated fat, specifically omega-3s and omega-6 fatty acids. These are considered good fatty acids that raise good cholesterol and prevent heart disease (source: *Very Well Fit*). Studies on post-menopausal women have found a 2g dose of pumpkin seed oil per day for 12 weeks can decrease blood pressure (source: *https://clinicaltrials.gov/ct2/show/NCT02727036*). Saturated fat content: 10.1g (per 100g), Sodium content: 0mg (per 100g), Sugar content: 0mg (per 100g).

Diverticulitis: Allowed on the high-fiber diet.

Histamine: Tolerated.

Lectins: High in lectins.

Oxalates: See "Pumpkin seeds"

Salicylates: See "Pumpkin seeds"

Pumpkin

- DASH: Fat: ✓ Sodium: ✓ Sugar: ✓
- Diverticulitis: Stage 1: ✗ Stage 2: 😐 Stage 3: ✓
- Histamine: ✗
- Lectin: ✗
- Oxalate: ✓
- Salicylates: ✓

DASH Diet (Hypertension): Allowed. Pumpkin contains vitamins A and C, both vital for good health (source: *BBC Good Food*). Saturated fat content: 0.1g (per 100g), Sodium content: 1 mg (per 100g), less than 1% daily value based on a 2,000 calorie diet, Sugar content: 2.8g (per 100g).

Diverticulitis: No solid foods can be eaten at stage one, the clear liquids diet. Test cautiously on the low-fiber diet.

Histamine: The respected site Fact vs Fitness puts pumpkin on their restricted list.

Lectins: Pumpkin is a source of lectins (source: *Functional Nutrition Library*). Peeling and deseeding help to reduce lectin content.

Oxalates: Canned pumpkins are thought to have a very low content, and raw pumpkins are negligible. Pumpkin seeds are different - see above.

Salicylates: Most reliable sources consider fresh and canned pumpkins low in salicylates, with analysis revealing .12 mg per 100 mg. However, some list pumpkins as containing a moderate level of salicylates. If you tolerate pumpkin well, you'll benefit from many nutrients like vitamins A, C, manganese, folate, potassium, calcium, and some B vitamins.

Pumpkin seeds

- DASH: Fat: ✓ Sodium: ✓ Sugar: ✓
- Diverticulitis: Stage 1: ✗ Stage 2: ✗ Stage 3: ✓
- Histamine: ✓
- Lectin: ✗
- Oxalate: 😐
- Salicylates: ✗

DASH Diet (Hypertension): Allowed. Pumpkin seeds are a healthy source of unsaturated fat (source: *BBC Good Food*). *Saturated fat content: 3.7g (per 100g), Sodium content: 18mg (per 100g), less than 1% daily value based on a 2,000 calorie diet, Sugar content: 0g (per 100g).*

Diverticulitis: No solid foods can be eaten at stage one, the clear liquids diet. Allowed on the high-fiber diet.

Histamine: Occasionally, we notice a reaction to pumpkin seeds. Most of the recognized sources say they are low in histamine. It also applies to pumpkin seed oil.

Lectins: High in lectins. To reduce lectin content, Precision Nutrition recommends soaking and cooking pumpkin seeds. This is because the highest concentration of lectins can be found in the seeds of plants (source: *Diagnosis Diet*).

Oxalates: Considerable debate. Consume in small portions. The website Kidney Dietitian notes: *"Pumpkin seeds (or "pepitas") are more than a treat in the fall! You can find pumpkin seeds year round. Add them to salads, oatmeal, yogurt or make your own low oxalate trail mix! 5 mg oxalate per 1/4 cup."*

Salicylates: Thought to contain a moderate amount of salicylates.

Quinoa

- DASH: Fat: ✓ Sodium: ✓ Sugar: ✓
- Diverticulitis: Stage 1: ✗ Stage 2: ✗ Stage 3: ✓
- Histamine: ✓
- Lectin: ✗
- Oxalate: ✗
- Salicylates: ✓

DASH Diet (Hypertension): Allowed. Add quinoa to your diet for a dose of healthy whole grains. *Saturated fat content: 0g (per 100g), Sodium content: 5 mg (per 100g) less than 1% daily value based on a 2,000 calorie diet, Sugar content: 0.9g (per 100g).*

Diverticulitis: No solid foods can be eaten at stage one, the clear liquids diet. Allowed on the high-fiber diet.

Histamine: A good gluten-free option.

Lectins: High in lectins. One to put on your 'avoid' list.

Oxalates: Thought to be high in oxalates. Approach with caution.

Salicylates: Quinoa is not only a whole protein, it's a versatile gluten-free and salicylate-free seed that can be ground into flour, used whole in stews, or even as a breakfast cereal.

Rabbit

- DASH: Fat: ✗ Sodium: ✓ Sugar: ✓
- Diverticulitis: Stage 1: ✗ Stage 2: ✓ Stage 3: ✗

- Histamine: ✓
- Lectin: ✓
- Oxalate: ✓
- Salicylates: ✓

DASH Diet (Hypertension): Rabbit is high in saturated fat, so it may not be the best protein choice for the DASH diet. *Saturated fat content: 2.5g (per 100g), Sodium content: 199 mg (per 100g) 9% daily value based on a 2,000 calorie diet, Sugar content: 0g (per 100g)* (source: *Fatsecret Platform API*).

Diverticulitis: No solid foods can be eaten at stage one, the clear liquids diet. Meat contains no fiber, so rabbit is allowed on a low-fiber diet.

Histamine: Organic, freshly cooked meat is typically safe.

Lectins: Thought to be low-lectin. Opt for grass-fed rabbits.

Oxalates: Low oxalate. However, eating large portions of meat can potentially increase the risk of kidney stones.

Salicylates: See "Meats"

Raclette cheese

- DASH: Fat: ✗ Sodium: ✗ Sugar: ✓
- Diverticulitis: Stage 1: ✗ Stage 2: ✓ Stage 3: ✗
- Histamine: ✗
- Lectin: ✓
- Oxalate: ✓
- Salicylates: ✓

A traditional Swiss melting cheese.

DASH Diet (Hypertension): High in saturated fat and sodium. Avoid. *Saturated fat content: 17.9g (per 100g), Sodium content: 551mg (per 100g), 24% daily value based on a 2,000 calorie diet, Sugar content: 0.5g (per 100g)* (source: *Fatsecret Platform API*).

Diverticulitis: No solid foods can be eaten at stage one, the clear liquids diet. Cheese contains no fiber, so they're allowed on a low-fiber diet.

Histamine: Avoid.

Lectins: It seems that most cheese from Switzerland is produced from A2 cow's milk (cows that originated in the Channel Islands and Southern France). If this is the case with raclette cheese, it's considered acceptable on a low lectin diet.

Oxalates: See cheeses. Thought to be low oxalate.

Salicylates: Most cheeses are thought to be very low in salicylates. Choose cheeses made from 100 percent grass-fed animals for the highest level of nutrients and avoid processed types that may contain salicylates and other potentially harmful ingredients.

Radish

- DASH: Fat: ✓ Sodium: ✓ Sugar: ✓
- Diverticulitis: Stage 1: ✗ Stage 2: ✗ Stage 3: ✓
- Histamine: ✓
- Lectin: ✓

- Oxalate: ✓
- Salicylates: ✗

DASH Diet (Hypertension): Allowed. Radishes are ripe with antioxidants that can help protect and promote heart health (source: *Real Simple*). *Saturated fat content: 0g (per 100g), Sodium content: 39mg (per 100g) 1% daily value based on a 2,000 calorie diet, Sugar content: 1.9g (per 100g).*

Diverticulitis: No solid foods can be eaten at stage one, the clear liquids diet. Allowed on the high-fiber diet.

Histamine: Low histamine and applies to red and white radishes.

Lectins: Falls under the cruciferous vegetable family (includes broccoli, kale, cabbage, radish etc.). These are considered low lectin and rich in vitamin C, folate and fiber.

Oxalates: White radish is considered to be low in oxalates, red radish is considered to be very low.

Salicylates: High in salicylates.

Raisins

- DASH: Fat: ✓ Sodium: ✓ Sugar: ✗
- Diverticulitis: Stage 1: ✗ Stage 2: ✗ Stage 3: ✓
- Histamine: ✓
- Lectin: 😐
- Oxalate: ✓
- Salicylates: ✗

DASH Diet (Hypertension): Raisins are high in sugar. Try to limit or avoid on the DASH diet. *Saturated fat content: 0.1g (per 100g), Sodium content: 11 mg (per 100g) less than 1% daily value based on a 2,000 calorie diet, Sugar content: 59g (per 100g).*

Diverticulitis: No solid foods can be eaten at stage one, the clear liquids diet. Allowed on the high-fiber diet.

Histamine: As long as there's no sulfur, you should find these are okay. However, most raisins have added sunflower oil.

Lectins: Raisins are dried grapes, and we know grapes contain moderate lectin content. Eat in moderation because of the high sugar content. Note that the nutrition content of grapes depends on how they are grown. For example, it's thought that grapes grown at a higher altitude are exposed to the sun. Hence, they contain higher levels of Polyphenols (anti-oxidants) (source: *Katherine Senko: Polyphenols in Wine*).

Oxalates: Low but not negligible.

Salicylates: Raisins are very high in salicylates, with some of the highest levels of any fruit analyzed by the American Dietetic Association.

Rapeseed oil (called canola oil in the US)

- DASH: Fat: ✗ Sodium: ✓ Sugar: ✓
- Diverticulitis: Stage 1: ✗ Stage 2: ✓ Stage 3: ✗
- Histamine: ✓
- Lectin: ✗
- Oxalate: ✓
- Salicylates: ✓

Known as *canola oil* in the U.S. and rapeseed oil in many other countries. Most often used as a cooking oil.

DASH Diet (Hypertension): Use in moderation because of the high saturated fat content. *Saturated fat content: 8g (per 100g), Sodium content: 0 mg (per 100g) 0% daily value based on a 2,000 calorie diet, Sugar content: 0g (per 100g).*

Diverticulitis: Allowed on the low-fiber diet, we suggest limiting rapeseed oil as it's not the healthiest.

Histamine: We've noticed it can cause inflammation. But you might well find it agrees with you.

Lectins: High in lectins. One to put on your 'avoid' list.

Oxalates: The site The VP Foundation notes all vegetable oils, including olive, canola, safflower, soy and margarine, are low oxalate.

Salicylates: Unlike peanut oil and olive oil, rapeseed oil contains only a negligible amount of salicylates. However, while some can tolerate canola oil well, it can lead to inflammation in others. Several animal studies have linked it to oxidative stress and increased inflammation. An Australian study published in *Lipids in Health and Disease* found that rats fed a diet that included 10 percent canola oil experienced increases in LDL ("bad") cholesterol and decreases in multiple antioxidants. The website *Food Can Make You Ill* provides a comprehensive breakdown of an Australian study (Anne R Swain et al. Salicylates in Food. Journal of the American Dietetic Association Vol. 85:8 1985). It notes; "*Margarine and processed rapeseed (canola), safflower, soya bean, sunflower oils, although low in salicylate, are likely to contain preservatives that may mimic salicylate reactions and are best avoided*".

Raspberry

- DASH: Fat: ✓ Sodium: ✓ Sugar: ✓
- Diverticulitis: Stage 1: ✗ Stage 2: ✗ Stage 3: ✓
- Histamine: ✗
- Lectin: ✓
- Oxalate: ✗
- Salicylates: ✗

Raspberries are a great source of vitamin C—just one cup provides over 50% of the daily vitamin C target!

DASH Diet (Hypertension): Allowed. Raspberries are one of the lowest sugar fruits. *Saturated fat content: 0g (per 100g), Sodium content: 1g (per 100g), less than 1% daily value based on a 2,000 calorie diet, Sugar content: 4.4g (per 100g).*

Diverticulitis: No solid foods can be eaten at stage one, the clear liquids diet. Allowed on the high-fiber diet.

Histamine: Avoid.

Lectins: Contains relatively low-lectins. It should be reasonably acceptable on a low-lectin diet in moderate quantities.

Oxalates: Considered to be high in oxalates. 100 g contains around 48 mg of oxalates, according to the University of Chicago. However, the Pain Spy Low Oxalate Foods List considers there to be 55 mg of oxalates in black raspberries and 15mg in red raspberries.

Salicylates: Raspberries are a significant source of salicylates. The website Allergy Link puts raspberries on its list of salicylate-containing foods that should be treated cautiously.

Red cabbage

- DASH: Fat: ✓ Sodium: ✓ Sugar: ✓
- Diverticulitis: Stage 1: ✗ Stage 2: ✗ Stage 3: ✓

- Histamine: ✓
- Lectin: ✓
- Oxalate: ✓
- Salicylates: ✓

One of the cabbage varieties.

DASH Diet (Hypertension): Allowed. Red cabbage is rich in antioxidants like anthocyanin that promote heart health (source: *BBC Good Food*). *Saturated fat content: 0g (per 100g), Sodium content: 27 mg (per 100g) 1% daily value based on a 2,000 calorie diet, Sugar content: 3.8g (per 100g).*

Diverticulitis: No solid foods can be eaten at stage one, the clear liquids diet. Allowed on the high-fiber diet.

Histamine: See more under "Cabbage".

Lectins: Thought to be low-lectin.

Oxalates: Thought to be low in oxalates.

Salicylates: Thankfully, cabbage is considered low in salicylates and versatile and cheap, even when purchasing organic. Plus, just a half-cup cooked provides about a third of your daily vitamin C requirements.

Red wine vinegar

- DASH: Fat: ✓ Sodium: ✓ Sugar: ✓
- Diverticulitis: Stage 1: ✗ Stage 2: ✓ Stage 3: ✗
- Histamine: ✗
- Lectin: ✓
- Oxalate: ✓
- Salicylates: ✗

DASH Diet (Hypertension): Allowed. Red wine vinegar contains powerful antioxidants that promote heart health (source: *Healthline*). *Saturated fat content: 0g (per 100g), Sodium content: 8mg (per 100g), 1% daily value based on a 2,000 calorie diet, Sugar content: 0g (per 100g)* (source: *Eat This Much*).

Diverticulitis: Contains no fiber, so they're allowed on the low-fiber diet.

Histamine: All vinegar is listed as high histamine apart from Apple Cider Vinegar. See other vinegars for more details.

Lectins: It's thought that all types of vinegar are tolerated on a low-lectin diet.

Oxalates: Thought to be low in oxalate. See other vinegars for more details.

Salicylates: High in salicylates with up to 1 mg per 100 mg.

Redcurrants

- DASH: Fat: ✓ Sodium: ✓ Sugar: ✗
- Diverticulitis: Stage 1: ✗ Stage 2: ✗ Stage 3: ✓
- Histamine: ✓
- Lectin: ✗
- Oxalate: ✗
- Salicylates: ✗

A member of the gooseberry family.

DASH Diet (Hypertension): Redcurrants are high in sugar. Try to avoid it. *Saturated fat content: 0.2 g (per 100g), Sodium content: 1 mg (per 100g) less than 1% daily value based on a 2,000 calorie diet, Sugar content: 7.4g (per 100g).*

Diverticulitis: No solid foods can be eaten at stage one, the clear liquids diet. Allowed on the high-fiber diet.

Histamine: Tolerated.

Lectins: As studies on redcurrants and lectins are limited, we recommend proceeding cautiously. Since gooseberries are related to currants, we think they could also be a source of lectins.

Oxalates: Winchester Hospital lists them as high and best avoided.

Salicylates: Very high in salicylates. Currants are among the highest salicylate foods.

Rhubarb
- DASH: Fat: ✓ Sodium: ✓ Sugar: ✓
- Diverticulitis: Stage 1: ✗ Stage 2: ✗ Stage 3: ✓
- Histamine: 😐
- Lectin: ✓
- Oxalate: ✗
- Salicylates: ✓

DASH Diet (Hypertension): Allowed. The high fiber content in rhubarb may benefit heart health (source: *Verywell Fit*). *Saturated fat content: 0.1g (per 100g), Sodium content: 4 mg (per 100g) less than 1% daily value based on a 2,000 calorie diet, Sugar content: 1.1g (per 100g).*

Diverticulitis: No solid foods can be eaten at stage one, the clear liquids diet. Allowed on the high-fiber diet.

Histamine: Test carefully.

Lectins: Contains very little lectin. It shouldn't cause any issues but test carefully.

Oxalates: Thought to contain massive amounts of oxalates. The food lists estimate between 541 mg and 800 mg per 100 grams, making it one of the most oxalate-loaded foods. This makes it one of our highest oxalate foods in this book. All of this means you'll sadly have to avoid rhubarb crumble on a low oxalate diet, but you could replace it with apple crumble.

Salicylates: Fresh rhubarb is thought to be low in salicylates. The website *Food Can Make You Ill* provides a comprehensive breakdown of an Australian study (Anne R Swain et al. Salicylates in Food. Journal of the American Dietetic Association Vol. 85:8 1985). It includes rhubarb in its 'low' list.

Rice
- DASH: Fat: ✓ Sodium: ✓ Sugar: ✓
- Diverticulitis: Stage 1: ✗ Stage 2: ✓ Stage 3: ✓
- Histamine: ✓
- Lectin: ✗
- Oxalate: 😐
- Salicylates: ✓

DASH Diet (Hypertension): Allowed. The DASH diet recommends several servings of whole grains per day. *Saturated fat content: 0.1g (per 100g), Sodium content: 1 mg (per 100g) less than 1% daily value based on a 2,000 calorie diet, Sugar content: 0.1g (per 100g).*

Diverticulitis: No solid foods can be eaten at stage one, the clear liquids diet. White rice is low in fiber. For a high-fiber diet, go for brown rice.

Histamine: Please note that whilst freshly cooked rice is what we are referring to here, pre-cooked packaged rice may have different histamine levels.

Lectins: Mixed opinion. One source points to no lectins in rice however, a study found lectins in rice (source: *Al Atalah B, De Vleesschauwer D, Xu J, Fouquaert E, Höfte M, Van Damme EJ. Transcriptional behavior of EUL-related rice lectins toward important abiotic and biotic stresses*). Other sources confirm that white rice contains fewer lectins than brown rice. It's recommended to use a pressure cooker to kill off lectins. It's thought that boiling rice also reduces lectin content.

Oxalates: Varies considerably depending on the rice. White rice has very low oxalate, but brown rice is thought to be moderate. Winchester Hospital qualifies wild rice as low oxalate. Black rice is high in oxalates.

Salicylates: Rice of all types is thought to contain trace amounts of salicylates.

Rice cakes

- DASH: Fat: ✓ Sodium: ✗ Sugar: ✓
- Diverticulitis: Stage 1: ✗ Stage 2: ✓ Stage 3: ✗
- Histamine: ✓
- Lectin: 😕
- Oxalate: 😕
- Salicylates: ✓

A snack food made from puffed rice.

DASH Diet (Hypertension): Thought to be high in sodium content. The amount of sodium varies by brand. Go for unsalted rice cakes. *Saturated fat content: 0.57g (per 100g), Sodium content: 326mg (per 100g), Sugar content: 0.88g (per 100g) (source: Fatsecret Platform API).*

Diverticulitis: No solid foods can be eaten at stage one, the clear liquids diet. Rice cakes are low in fiber, so they're allowed on a low-fiber diet.

Histamine: Tolerated.

Lectins: As above, there is a mixed opinion on the consumption of rice.

Oxalates: See Rice.

Salicylates: While rice contains very little or no salicylates, rice cakes typically contain other ingredients that are not or that may have a negative impact on health, like sugars and artificial colorings. Look for non-GMO, organic options and check individual ingredients.

Rice milk

- DASH: Fat: ✓ Sodium: ✓ Sugar: ✗
- Diverticulitis: Stage 1: ✗ Stage 2: ✓ Stage 3: ✗
- Histamine: 😕
- Lectin: 😕
- Oxalate: 😕
- Salicylates: ✓

DASH Diet (Hypertension): Rice milk contains all the healthy nutrients that rice does. However, it lacks some protein that other milk choices like cow and soy provide (source: *Healthline*). *Saturated fat content: 0g (per 100g), Sodium content: 39 mg (per 100g), 1% daily value based on a 2,000 calorie diet, Sugar content: 5g (per 100g).*

Diverticulitis: Low in fiber, so allowed on the low-fiber diet.

Histamine: Watch out for added ingredients in rice milk. As a rule of thumb, the few ingredients, the better.

Lectins: As above, there is a mixed opinion on rice consumption. Test carefully.

Oxalates: See Rice.

Salicylates: Generally, rice milk is low in salicylates; however, you'll need to check the individual ingredients. For example, some include canola, safflower or sunflower oils, flavorings, and other additives. Important note: Be aware that non-animal milk often used in coffee shops like almond and coconut milk, has a high level of salicylates. Rice milk will hopefully work better for you but can be higher in sugar.

Rice noodles

- DASH: Fat: ✓ Sodium: ✓ Sugar: ✓
- Diverticulitis: Stage 1: ✗ Stage 2: ✓ Stage 3: ✗
- Histamine: ✓
- Lectin: ✗
- Oxalate: 😐
- Salicylates: ✓

DASH Diet (Hypertension): Allowed. Rice noodles can be a great source of complex carbohydrates, especially for those who are gluten-free (source: *Verywell Fit*). *Saturated fat content: 0g (per 100g), Sodium content: 19 mg (per 100g), less than 1% daily value based on a 2,000 calorie diet, Sugar content: 0g (per 100g).*

Diverticulitis: No solid foods can be eaten at stage one, the clear liquids diet. Low in fiber, so allowed on the low-fiber diet.

Histamine: Tolerated.

Lectins: Made from rice flour which is high in lectins. Best to avoid.

Oxalates: See Rice.

Salicylates: Typically low in salicylates, but again, it's important to check individual ingredients.

Ricotta cheese

- DASH: Fat: ✗ Sodium: ✓ Sugar: ✓
- Diverticulitis: Stage 1: ✗ Stage 2: ✓ Stage 3: ✗
- Histamine: 😐
- Lectin: 😐
- Oxalate: ✓
- Salicylates: ✓

DASH Diet (Hypertension): High in saturated fat. Try to limit or avoid on the DASH diet. *Saturated fat content: 8g (per 100g), Sodium content: 84 mg (per 100g) 3% daily value based on a 2,000 calorie diet, Sugar content: 0.3g (per 100g).*

Diverticulitis: No solid foods can be eaten at stage one, the clear liquids diet. Cheese contains no fiber, so they're allowed on a low-fiber diet.

Histamine: Tends to be one of the best-tolerated cheeses. As this is a soft cheese, it may be a better option for you.

Lectins: Depends on the milk as ricotta cheese can be made from cow, sheep, goat or water buffalo's milk (source: *Bon Appetit*). Avoid ricotta cheese made from cow's milk.

Oxalates: Cheeses are generally considered low in oxalate.

Salicylates: Most cheeses are thought to be very low in salicylates.

Choose ricotta cheese made from 100 percent grass-fed animals for the highest level of nutrients and avoid processed types containing salicylates and other potentially harmful ingredients.

Rooibos tea

- DASH: Fat: ✓ Sodium: ✓ Sugar: ✓
- Diverticulitis: Stage 1: ✓ Stage 2: ✓ Stage 3: ✗
- Histamine: ✓
- Lectin: ✓
- Oxalate: ✓
- Salicylates: ✗

DASH Diet (Hypertension): Allowed on the DASH diet. A study suggested that rooibos tea may act as a natural blood pressure reducer (source: *WebMD*). Saturated fat content: 0g (per 100g), Sodium content: 0g (per 100g), 0% daily value based on a 2,000 calorie diet, Sugar content: 0g (per 100g) (source: *WebMD*).

Diverticulitis: Tea with no milk or cream is allowed at stage one, the clear liquid diet. Also allowed on the low-fiber diet.

Histamine: Tolerated.

Lectins: It's thought that tea is acceptable on a low-lectin diet.

Oxalates: Just 0.55-1.06 mg of oxalate per cup based on steep time (source: *Pubmed, National Library of Medicine*). The site lowoxalateinfo.com notes: "Rooibos is the first low oxalate tea I have found that both tastes great and is full-bodied enough to enjoy hot with cream."

Salicylates: Very high in salicylates.

Roquefort cheese

- DASH: Fat: ✗ Sodium: ✗ Sugar: ✓
- Diverticulitis: Stage 1: ✗ Stage 2: ✓ Stage 3: ✗
- Histamine: 😐
- Lectin: 😐
- Oxalate: ✓
- Salicylates: ✓

A type of blue cheese made from sheep's milk.

DASH Diet (Hypertension): High in saturated fat and sodium. Avoid. *Saturated fat content: 19.3g (per 100g), Sodium content: 1809mg (per 100g) 79% daily value based on a 2,000 calorie diet, Sugar content: 0g (per 100g).*

Diverticulitis: No solid foods can be eaten at stage one, the clear liquids diet. Cheese contains no fiber, so they're allowed on the low-fiber diet.

Histamine: Test carefully.

Lectins: Cheese acquires lectins from the molds that grow within it (source: *Understanding Arthritis, The Clinical Way Forward by W. Fox, D. Freed*). Test carefully as molds are used in Roquefort production.

Oxalates: Cheeses are thought to be low oxalate.

Salicylates: Most cheeses are thought to be very low in salicylates. Choose Roquefort made from 100 percent grass-fed animals for the highest level of nutrients and avoid processed types that may contain salicylates and other potentially harmful ingredients.

Rosemary

- DASH: Fat: ✗ Sodium: ✓ Sugar: ✓
- Diverticulitis: Stage 1: ✗ Stage 2: 😐 Stage 3: ✓
- Histamine: ✓
- Lectin: ✓
- Oxalate: ✓
- Salicylates: ✗

DASH Diet (Hypertension): Allowed. Rosemary is rich in antioxidants that may help improve blood circulation (source: *Flushing Hospital*). *Saturated fat content: 2.8g (per 100g), Sodium content: 26mg (per 100g) 1% daily value based on a 2,000 calorie diet, Sugar content: 0g (per 100g).*

Diverticulitis: Test cautiously on a low-fiber diet.

Histamine: Tolerated.

Lectins: Acceptable.

Oxalates: Low in oxalates.

Salicylates: Very high in salicylates.

Rum

- DASH: Fat: ✓ Sodium: ✓ Sugar: ✓
- Diverticulitis: Stage 1: ✗ Stage 2: ✗ Stage 3: ✗
- Histamine: ✗
- Lectin: 😐
- Oxalate: ✓
- Salicylates: ✗

A distilled spirit made from fermented sugar (source: *Vine Pair*).

DASH Diet (Hypertension): Limit alcoholic beverages. *Saturated fat content: 0g (per 100g), Sodium content: 1 mg (per 100g), less than 1% daily value based on a 2,000 calorie diet, Sugar content: 0g (per 100g).*

Diverticulitis: See alcohol.

Histamine: Alcohol is high in histamine, and please check other notes on alcohol in this book. We find that some alcohols are slightly less inflammatory than others. Rum suits some better but is high histamine all the same.

Lectins: As studies on rum and lectins are limited, we recommend proceeding cautiously.

Oxalates: See alcohol.

Salicylates: Alcoholic beverages like rum contain a high level of salicylates.

Rye

- DASH: Fat: ✓ Sodium: ✓ Sugar: ✓
- Diverticulitis: Stage 1: ✗ Stage 2: ✗ Stage 3: ✓
- Histamine: 😐
- Lectin: ✗
- Oxalate: ✗
- Salicylates: ✓

DASH Diet (Hypertension): Rye bread is a nutritious choice for a daily serving of grains. *Saturated fat content: 0.6g (per 100g), Sodium content: 603 mg (per 100g) 25% daily value based on a 2,000 calorie diet, Sugar content: 3.9 g (per 100g).*

Diverticulitis: No solid foods can be eaten at stage one, the clear liquids diet. Rye is a whole grain that is a great source of fiber.

Histamine: Test carefully.

Lectins: A cereal grain high in lectins. One to put on your 'avoid' list. Avoid rye foods, such as rye bread, crackers, beer and whiskey (source: *The Spruce Eats*).

Oxalates: Rye flour is moderate to high in oxalates. The unprocessed grain is very high, with at least 15.0 mg per 100 g (source: *Urinary Stones Food List*).

Salicylates: Rye contains little if any salicylates; however if you are gluten intolerant, be aware that it is not gluten-free.

Sage

- DASH: Fat: ✗ Sodium: ✓ Sugar: ✓
- Diverticulitis: Stage 1: ✓ Stage 2: ✓ Stage 3: ✗
- Histamine: ✓
- Lectin: ✓
- Oxalate: ✓
- Salicylates: ✗

DASH Diet (Hypertension): Sage is a herb loaded with antioxidants. Use it to spruce up dishes with some added flavor. *Saturated fat content: 7.03g (per 100g), Sodium content: 11mg (per 100g), less than 1% daily value based on a 2,000 calorie diet, Sugar content: 1.7g (per 100g).*

Diverticulitis: Very low in fiber. Allowed on the low-fiber diet.

Histamine: Tolerated.

Lectins: Tolerated.

Oxalates: UPMC lists them as low oxalate.

Salicylates: High in salicylates.

Salami

- DASH: Fat: ✗ Sodium: ✗ Sugar: ✓

- Diverticulitis: Stage 1: ✗ Stage 2: ✓ Stage 3: ✗
- Histamine: ✗
- Lectin: ✓
- Oxalate: ✓
- Salicylates: ✗

A cured sausage.

DASH Diet (Hypertension): High in saturated fat and sodium. Try to limit or avoid. *Saturated fat content: 9 g (per 100g), Sodium content: 1,740 mg (per 100g) 72% daily value based on a 2,000 calorie diet, Sugar content: 1g (per 100g).*

Diverticulitis: No solid foods can be eaten at stage one, the clear liquids diet. Meat contains no fiber, so salami is allowed on the low-fiber diet.

Histamine: Cured meats should be avoided, and unfortunately, salami comes into this category. Cured meats are poor for health and high in histamine.

Lectins: As meats are generally low in lectins, dry-cured meats such as salami are permitted on a low-lectin diet. Ensure the salami is made from grass-fed meat.

Oxalates: Low oxalate. However, eating large portions of meat can potentially increase the risk of kidney stones. Cured meats are generally considered bad for your health.

Salicylates: See "Dry-cured meats"

Salmon

- DASH: Fat: ✗ Sodium: ✓ Sugar: ✓
- Diverticulitis: Stage 1: ✗ Stage 2: ✓ Stage 3: ✗
- Histamine: ✗
- Lectin: ✓
- Oxalate: ✓
- Salicylates: ✓

DASH Diet (Hypertension): Salmon is a great source of omega-3 fatty acids and potassium, which can help maintain blood pressure and contribute to heart health (source: *Safe Beat*). *Saturated fat content: 3.1g (per 100g), Sodium content: 59 mg (per 100g) 2% daily value based on a 2,000 calorie diet, Sugar content: 0g (per 100g).*

Diverticulitis: No solid foods can be eaten at stage one, the clear liquids diet. Seafood contains no fiber, so salmon is allowed on a low-fiber diet.

Histamine: Salmon deserves some special comments here because while all fish is high in histamine levels, salmon is one that, if caught and frozen quickly, is tolerated much more effectively. We have found some good salmon brands which deliver frozen. Wild-caught and organic are best.

Lectins: Allowed on a low-lectin diet. For a healthier option, opt for wild-caught salmon. These are lower in calories and have higher potassium levels and other minerals (source: *Wild For Salmon*).

Oxalates: Good news, salmon is considered to have little or no oxalates, like most fish.

Salicylates: Fish contains no to only trace amounts of salicylates, according to most reliable sources.

Sauerkraut

- DASH: Fat: ✓ Sodium: ✗ Sugar: ✓
- Diverticulitis: Stage 1: ✗ Stage 2: ✗ Stage 3: ✓

- Histamine: ✗
- Lectin: ✓
- Oxalate: ✓
- Salicylates: ✗

DASH Diet (Hypertension): Sauerkraut is high in sodium, but it is also full of healthy vitamins and minerals. Enjoy in moderation. *Saturated fat content: 0g (per 100g), Sodium content: 661 mg (per 100g), 27% daily value based on a 2,000 calorie diet, Sugar content: 1.8g (per 100g).*

Diverticulitis: No solid foods can be eaten at stage one, the clear liquids diet. Sauerkraut is high in fiber. Allowed on the high-fiber diet.

Histamine: Very high in histamine.

Lectins: Raw sauerkraut is thought to be low-lectin.

Oxalates: Low, you can have it in any quantity, although you should still combine it with calcium.

Salicylates: Very high in salicylates.

Sausages of all kinds

- DASH: Fat: ✗ Sodium: ✗ Sugar: N/A
- Diverticulitis: Stage 1: ✗ Stage 2: ✓ Stage 3: ✗
- Histamine: ✗
- Lectin: ✓
- Oxalate: ✓
- Salicylates: ✗

DASH Diet (Hypertension): Avoid. Sausage is processed meat high in saturated fat and sodium content. If you must eat meat, go for lean and low-fat meat. *Saturated fat content: 11g (per 100g), Sodium content: 731mg (per 100g) 30% daily value based on a 2,000 calorie diet, Sugar content: N/A.*

Diverticulitis: No solid foods can be eaten at stage one, the clear liquids diet. Meat contains no fiber, so sausages are allowed on the low-fiber diet.

Histamine: Avoid.

Lectins: Fresh sausages without high lectin ingredients are permitted (source: *US Wellness Meats*). Opt for grass-fed sausages. Sausages can have other added ingredients, so check carefully.

Oxalates: See meat.

Salicylates: While most meats are free of salicylates, sausage contains spices and other flavorings that make it best to avoid for those who are sensitive.

Savoy cabbage

- DASH: Fat: ✓ Sodium: ✓ Sugar: ✓
- Diverticulitis: Stage 1: ✗ Stage 2: ✗ Stage 3: ✓
- Histamine: 🤔
- Lectin: ✓
- Oxalate: ✓
- Salicylates: ✓

One of the cabbage varieties. Rich in vitamin B6 and folate, which are essential nutrients.

DASH Diet (Hypertension): Include cabbage in your diet to reach 4-5 servings of vegetables a day. *Saturated fat content: 0g (per 100g), Sodium content: 28 mg (per 100g) 1% daily value based on a 2,000 calorie diet, Sugar content: 2.3g (per 100g).*

Diverticulitis: No solid foods can be eaten at stage one, the clear liquids diet. Allowed on the high-fiber diet.

Histamine: Test carefully.

Lectins: Thought to be low-lectin.

Oxalates: Thought to be low in oxalates.

Salicylates: Thankfully, cabbage is considered low in salicylates and versatile and cheap, even when purchasing organic. Plus, just a half-cup cooked provides about a third of your daily vitamin C requirements. As always, test carefully, but cabbage is one of our low-salicylate staples.

Schnapps

- DASH: Fat: ✓ Sodium: ✓ Sugar: ✓
- Diverticulitis: Stage 1: ✗ Stage 2: ✗ Stage 3: ✗
- Histamine: ✗
- Lectin: 😕
- Oxalate: ✓
- Salicylates: ✗

A type of alcohol.

DASH Diet (Hypertension): The above nutritional values are based on Peach Schnapps from Calorie Counter's website. The sugar content varies depending on the flavor. Schnapps is thought to be high in calories. As Schnapps are a type of alcohol, watch consumption. *Saturated fat content: 0g (per 100g), Sodium content: 3mg (per 100g), Sugar content: 4g (per 100g).*

Diverticulitis: See 'Alcohol'

Histamine: See "Alcohol"

Lectins: As studies on schnapps and lectins are limited, we recommend proceeding cautiously.

Oxalates: See "Alcohol"

Salicylates: Alcoholic beverages tend to contain a high level of salicylates. See "Alcohol" for more details.

Seafood

- DASH: Fat: ✓ Sodium: ✓ Sugar: N/A
- Diverticulitis: Stage 1: ✗ Stage 2: ✓ Stage 3: ✗
- Histamine: ✗
- Lectin: 😕
- Oxalate: ✓
- Salicylates: ✓

DASH Diet (Hypertension): Check individual seafood for specific nutritional values. *Saturated fat content: 1.9g (per 100g), Sodium content: 117 mg (per 100g), 4% daily value based on a 2,000 calorie diet, Sugar content: N/A.*

Diverticulitis: No solid foods can be eaten at stage one, the clear liquids diet. Seafood contains no fiber, so it is allowed on a low-fiber diet.

Histamine: All seafood except freshly caught and frozen we list as high histamine. Fish also increases in histamine extraordinarily quickly. Certain fish can be okay if caught fresh and then frozen quickly after catching them. Fish freshly caught within an hour or frozen within an hour may well be better tolerated. Any fish in fishmongers or smoked should be avoided.

Lectins: Depends on the type. Wild-caught seafood is thought to be low in lectin.

Oxalates: Low.

Salicylates: Fish contains no to only trace amounts of salicylates, according to most reliable sources.

Seaweed

- DASH: Fat: ✓ Sodium: ✓ Sugar: ✓
- Diverticulitis: Stage 1: ✗ Stage 2: ✗ Stage 3: ✓
- Histamine: ✗
- Lectin: ✓
- Oxalate: 😕
- Salicylates: ✗

DASH Diet (Hypertension): Seaweed is a great source of dietary iodine. Eat dried seaweed as a healthy snack or add fresh seaweed to cooked dishes. *Saturated fat content: 0.1g (per 100g), Sodium content: 102 mg (per 100g) 4% daily value based on a 2,000 calorie diet, Sugar content: 3g (per 100g).*

Diverticulitis: No solid foods can be eaten at stage one, the clear liquids diet. An excellent source of fiber, so allowed on the high-fiber diet.

Histamine: Avoid.

Lectins: Thought to be low-lectin. Health Canal's website refers to bladderwrack seaweed as a *"natural lectin blocker"*.

Oxalates: Varies. Some kinds are thought to prevent the formation of calcium oxalate kidney stones. Research published in the Journal of Functional Foods shows that sulphated polysaccharides (SPSs) from various seaweeds possess broad-spectrum therapeutic and biomedical properties that significantly inhibit these stones.

Salicylates: Very high in salicylates.

Sesame

- DASH: Fat: ✗ Sodium: ✓ Sugar: ✓
- Diverticulitis: Stage 1: ✗ Stage 2: ✗ Stage 3: ✓
- Histamine: ✓
- Lectin: ✗
- Oxalate: ✗
- Salicylates: 😕

DASH Diet (Hypertension): Sesame seeds are a rich source of protein and calcium. Consume in moderation as part of a healthy diet (source: *WebMD*). *Saturated fat content: 7g (per 100g), Sodium content: 11 mg (per 100g) less than 1% daily value based on a 2,000 calorie diet, Sugar content: 0.3g (per 100g).*

Diverticulitis: No solid foods can be eaten at stage one, the clear liquids diet. Allowed on the high-fiber diet.

Histamine: Sesame seeds also seem to be tolerated.

Lectins: Sesame is a source of lectins (source: *Functional Nutrition Library*).

Oxalates: 15.0 mg & up per 100 g, very high oxalate content (source: *Urinary Stones - The Oxalate Content Of Food*).

Salicylates: There is a distinction here between sesame seeds and sesame oil. Sesame seeds are thought to be lowish in salicylates. However, sesame oil contains a higher amount and should be limited or avoided.

Sheep's milk, sheep milk

- DASH: Fat: ✗ Sodium: ✓ Sugar: ✓
- Diverticulitis: Stage 1: ✗ Stage 2: ✓ Stage 3: ✗
- Histamine: ✓
- Lectin: ✓
- Oxalate: ✓
- Salicylates: ✓

Sheep's milk is an alternative to cow's, full of nutrients and protein. It is commonly used in some types of cheeses, such as feta cheese.

DASH Diet (Hypertension): Consume in moderation because of the high-fat content.

Diverticulitis: Sheep milk contains no fiber, so they're allowed on the low-fiber diet.

Histamine: Tolerated.

Lectins: Tolerated on a low-lectin diet. Sheep milk is often digested easier than normal dairy as it contains more A2 beta-casein proteins (source: *Parsley Health*).

Oxalates: See "Milk"

Salicylates: See "Milk" - generally a good option.

Shellfish

- DASH: Fat: ✓ Sodium: ✓ Sugar: N/A
- Diverticulitis: Stage 1: ✗ Stage 2: ✓ Stage 3: ✗
- Histamine: ✗
- Lectin: ✗
- Oxalate: ✓
- Salicylates: ✓

See *bivalves*.

DASH Diet (Hypertension): Allowed. *Saturated fat content: 0.1g (per 100g), Sodium content: 111 mg (per 100g) 4% daily value based on a 2,000 calorie diet, Sugar content: N/A.*

Diverticulitis: No solid foods can be eaten at stage one, the clear liquids diet. Seafood contains no fiber, so shellfish is allowed on the low-fiber diet.

Histamine: See comments on fish and seafood.

Lectins: A source of lectins. One to put on your 'avoid' list (source: *Live Pain Free Cookbook by Jesse Cannone*).

Oxalates: Low, as per seafood in general.

Salicylates: Fish is normally fine. See "Fish" and "Bivalves" and the note below under "Shrimp"

Shrimp

- DASH: Fat: ✓ Sodium: ✓ Sugar: ✓
- Diverticulitis: Stage 1: ✗ Stage 2: ✓ Stage 3: ✗
- Histamine: ✗
- Lectin: ✗
- Oxalate: ✓
- Salicylates: ✓

Also referred to as *prawns*.

DASH Diet (Hypertension): Allowed. Also, a great source of protein. *Saturated fat content: 0.1g (per 100g), Sodium content: 111 mg (per 100g), 4% daily value based on a 2,000 calorie diet, Sugar content: 0g (per 100g).*

Diverticulitis: No solid foods can be eaten at stage one, the clear liquids diet. Seafood contains no fiber, so shrimp is allowed on a low-fiber diet.

Histamine: Avoid.

Lectins: Seven groups of lectins have been found in shrimp (source: *Wang XW, Wang JX. Diversity and multiple functions of lectins in shrimp immunity. Dev Comp Immunol*). While we have not found a conclusive answer to the shrimp content in lectin, we believe it is best to avoid or approach cautiously.

Oxalates: Low, as per seafood in general.

Salicylates: Be aware that canned shrimp and/or shrimp sprayed with sulfites will contain a moderate to a high amount of salicylates. Avoid fried shrimp which typically contain a high level. See "Prawns" for another important note.

Smoked fish

- DASH: Fat: ✓ Sodium: ✗ Sugar: ✓
- Diverticulitis: Stage 1: ✗ Stage 2: ✓ Stage 3: ✗
- Histamine: ✗
- Lectin: ✓
- Oxalate: ✓
- Salicylates: ✗

DASH Diet (Hypertension): High in sodium. Avoid all things smoked as salt is used in the smoking process. *Saturated fat content: 0.9g (per 100g), Sodium content: 780mg (per 100g), 34% daily value based on a 2,000 calorie diet, Sugar content: 0g (per 100g)* (source: *Fatsecret Platform API*).

Diverticulitis: No solid foods can be eaten at stage one, the clear liquids diet. Seafood contains no fiber, so smoked fish is allowed on the low-fiber diet.

Histamine: Avoid.

Lectins: If wild-caught, then acceptable on a low-lectin diet.

Oxalates: See "fish".

Salicylates: Avoid processed fish.

Smoked meat

- DASH: Fat: ✓ Sodium: ✗ Sugar: ✓

- Diverticulitis: Stage 1: ✗ Stage 2: ✓ Stage 3: ✗
- Histamine: ✗
- Lectin: ✓
- Oxalate: ✓
- Salicylates: ✗

DASH Diet (Hypertension): Smoked meat includes sausages, bacon and ham, to name a few. Avoid all things smoked as salt is used in the smoking process. The National Cancer Institute notes a link between prostate, colon, rectal and pancreatic cancer and an increased intake of smoked meats. *Saturated fat content: 0.9g (per 100g), Sodium content: 908.4mg (per 100g), 38% daily value based on a 2,000 calorie diet, Sugar content: 0g (per 100g)* (source: *Nutritionix*).

Diverticulitis: No solid foods can be eaten at stage one, the clear liquids diet. Meat contains no fiber, so it is allowed on a low-fiber diet.

Histamine: Avoid.

Lectins: Allowed but ensure these are grass-fed.

Oxalates: Low oxalate. However, eating large portions of meat can potentially increase the risk of kidney stones.

Salicylates: While meats generally are free of salicylates, smoked meats typically contain a higher amount.

Snow peas

- DASH: Fat: ✓ Sodium: ✓ Sugar: ✗
- Diverticulitis: Stage 1: ✗ Stage 2: ✗ Stage 3: ✓
- Histamine: 😐
- Lectin: 😐
- Oxalate: ✓
- Salicylates: 😐

Also known as *Chinese pea pods*. Rich in fiber and iron, they also contain heart-healthy nutrients like potassium and calcium (source: *BBC Good Food*).

DASH Diet (Hypertension): Watch the sugar content.

Diverticulitis: No solid foods can be eaten at stage one, the clear liquids diet. Allowed on the high-fiber diet.

Histamine: See "green peas".

Lectins: Mixed opinion. Some say these contain low levels of lectin and are safe to eat. However, Dr Cordain mentioned on The Paleo Diet's website that consuming peas *"may still interfere with normal gut nutrient absorption"*. Limit consumption and test carefully.

Oxalates: See "green peas".

Salicylates: May contain a higher level of salicylates. Test carefully.

Soft cheese

- DASH:
  - Brie: Fat: ✗ Sodium: ✗ Sugar: ✓
  - Camembert: Fat: 😐 Sodium: 😐 Sugar: ✓
- Diverticulitis: Stage 1: ✗ Stage 2: ✓ Stage 3: ✗

- Histamine: 😬
- Lectin: 😬
- Oxalate: ✓
- Salicylates: ✓

Soft cheese typically includes feta, brie, ricotta, cream cheese, mozzarella and cottage cheese to name a few.

DASH Diet (Hypertension): Depends on the type of soft cheese. See the nutritional values for feta, cream cheese, roquefort and ricotta in this food list. **Brie**: *Saturated fat content: 17g (per 100g), Sodium content: 629 mg (per 100g), 26% daily value based on a 2,000 calorie diet, Sugar content: 0.5g (per 100g).* **Camembert**: *Saturated fat content: 15g (per 100g), Sodium content: 842mg (per 100g), 35% daily value based on a 2,000 calorie diet, Sugar content: 0.5g (per 100g).* Avoid brie and camembert as these are high in saturated fat and sodium. Cleveland Clinic recommends going for naturally low-sodium cheese such as Swiss, goat, brick ricotta and fresh mozzarella if you want cheese.

Diverticulitis: No solid foods can be eaten at stage one, the clear liquids diet. Cheese contains no fiber, so they're allowed on a low-fiber diet.

Histamine: See comments under 'Cheese'.

Lectins: Lectin content depends on the type of soft cheese. For example, Feta is considered low-lectin if made with sheep or goat's milk, and cottage cheese should be avoided, according to some sources. Some sources claim that very high-fat dairy products such as soft cheeses are low in casein and therefore low in lectin. Other sources mention all dairy products contain casein and should be avoided. Test carefully.

Oxalates: See comments under 'Cheese'.

Salicylates: Most cheeses are thought to be very low in salicylates. Choose cheeses made from 100 percent grass-fed animals for the highest level of nutrients and avoid processed types that may contain salicylates and other potentially harmful ingredients.

Sour cream

- DASH: Fat: ✗ Sodium: ✓ Sugar: ✓
- Diverticulitis: Stage 1: ✗ Stage 2: ✓ Stage 3: ✗
- Histamine: 😬
- Lectin: 😬
- Oxalate: ✓
- Salicylates: ✓

DASH Diet (Hypertension): High in saturated fat, so try to limit or avoid on the DASH diet. *Saturated fat content: 12g (per 100g), Sodium content: 80 mg (per 100g), 3% daily value based on a 2,000 calorie diet, Sugar content: 2.9g (per 100g).*

Diverticulitis: No solid foods can be eaten at stage one, the clear liquids diet. Sour cream contains no fiber, so it is allowed on the low-fiber diet.

Histamine: Test carefully.

Lectins: Some sources claim that very high fat dairy products such as sour cream are low in casein and therefore low in lectin. Other sources mention all dairy products contain casein and should be avoided. Test carefully.

Oxalates: Sour cream is a good choice for people on a low oxalate diet. The University of Virginia Digestive Health Center advises: "*Eat plenty of calcium-rich foods. Calcium binds to oxalate so that it isn't absorbed into your blood and cannot reach your kidneys. Dairy is free of oxalate and high in calcium, so it is an ideal choice. Choose skim, low fat, or* full fat versions depending on your weight goals. If you are lactose intolerant, look for lactose-free dairy such as Lactaid brand, or eat yogurt or kefir instead. "

Salicylates: Sour cream is low in salicylates; however, it's important to check for any added ingredients that may contain a higher level.

Soy (soybeans, soy flour)

- DASH: Fat: ✓ Sodium: ✗ Sugar: ✓
- Diverticulitis: Stage 1: ✗ Stage 2: ✗ Stage 3: ✓
- Histamine: ✗
- Lectin: ✗
- Oxalate: ✗
- Salicylates: ✗

DASH Diet (Hypertension): Soy is a protein rich food that can often replace animal protein products in a diet. However, it can be high in sodium, so try to limit or avoid on the DASH diet. *Saturated fat content: 0.4g (per 100g), Sodium content: 1,005 mg (per 100g), 41% daily value based on a 2,000 calorie diet, Sugar content: 0g (per 100g).*

Diverticulitis: No solid foods can be eaten at stage one, the clear liquids diet. Allowed on the high-fiber diet.

Histamine: Includes soy milk, soya milk, and other soy drinks .

Lectins: Soy beans are high in lectins. One to put in your 'avoid' list. According to the Food Chemistry Journal Volume 39, Issue 3, 1991, the amount of lectin in soy flour depends on the processing method used. Soy flour made from raw seeds contained the highest level of lectins. Successful attempts have been made to remove lectins from soybean flour using a bio-separation technique (source: *S. Bajpai et al. / Food Chemistry 89 (2005) 497-501*) but as these techniques cannot easily be performed in the kitchen, it's best to avoid.

Oxalates: Potentially high in oxalate depending on the soy product. Soy flour is thought to be high in oxalates. Approach each individual soy product carefully. Website WebMD notes; *"Products made from soybeans are excellent sources of protein and other nutrients, especially for people on a plant-based diet. However, they are also high in oxalates."*

Salicylates: An excellent source of protein that makes it especially ideal for anyone on a plant-based diet, soy contains negligible salicylates. There's a big but coming though. The website Food Can Make You Ill notes; *"Margarine and processed rapeseed (canola), safflower, soya bean, sunflower oils although low in salicylate are likely to contain preservatives that may mimic salicylate reactions and are best avoided."*

Soy sauce

- DASH: Fat: ✓ Sodium: ✗ Sugar: ✓
- Diverticulitis: Stage 1: ✗ Stage 2: ✓ Stage 3: ✗
- Histamine: ✗
- Lectin: ✗
- Oxalate: 🤔
- Salicylates: ✗

DASH Diet (Hypertension): Generally high in sodium. Try to limit or avoid on the DASH diet. *Saturated fat content: 0.1g (per 100g), Sodium content: 5,493 mg (per 100g), 228% daily value based on a 2,000 calorie diet, Sugar content: 0.4g (per 100g).*

Diverticulitis: Very low in fiber, so allowed on the low-fiber diet.

Histamine: Avoid.

Lectins: High in lectins. One to put on your 'avoid' list. See soy above.

Oxalates: Approach all soy products with caution. The good news is that soy sauce may be lower in oxalate than other soy products, such as soy flour.

Salicylates: Provided it is free of spices and other additives, soy sauce is low in salicylates. There's a big but coming though. The website *Food Can Make You Ill* notes; "*Margarine and processed rapeseed (canola), safflower, soya bean, sunflower oils, although low in salicylate, are likely to contain preservatives that may mimic salicylate reactions and are best avoided.*"

Sparkling wine
- DASH: Fat: ✓ Sodium: ✓ Sugar: ✓
- Diverticulitis: Stage 1: ✗ Stage 2: ✗ Stage 3: ✗
- Histamine: ✗
- Lectin: 😕
- Oxalate: ✓
- Salicylates: ✗

DASH Diet (Hypertension): Drink alcohol sparingly on the DASH diet. You don't have to eliminate alcohol completely although limiting consumption is good. *Saturated fat content: 0g (per 100g), Sodium content: 5mg (per 100g), less than 1% daily value based on a 2,000 calorie diet, Sugar content: 0.79g (per 100g)* (source: *Fatsecret Platform API*).

Diverticulitis: See alcohol.

Histamine: Avoid. More in the 'Alcohol' section.

Lectins: Lectin content should depend on the type of sparkling wine. Test carefully. We know that red wine contains high levels of Polyphenols (antioxidants) compared to other types of wine (including white wine). Some experts permit drinking wine high in Polyphenols (in moderation) on a low-lectin diet. Note that the nutrition content of red wine depends on how the grapes are grown. For example, it's thought that grapes grown at a higher altitude have greater exposure to the sun so they contain higher levels of Polyphenols (source: *Katherine Senko: Polyphenols in Wine*).

Oxalates: See alcohol.

Salicylates: Alcoholic beverages contain a high level of salicylates. See "alcohol" for more details. Sparkling wine is thought by some to be high.

Spelt
- DASH: Fat: ✓ Sodium: ✓ Sugar: ✗
- Diverticulitis: Stage 1: ✗ Stage 2: ✗ Stage 3: ✓
- Histamine: ✓
- Lectin: ✗
- Oxalate: 😕
- Salicylates: ✓

A type of grain similar to wheat. Fun fact: Spelt was one of the first grains to be used to make bread.

DASH Diet (Hypertension): Include as one of your whole grain servings of the day. *Saturated fat content: 0.4g (per 100g), Sodium content: 8 mg (per 100g), less than 1% daily value based on a 2,000 calorie diet, Sugar content: 7g (per 100g).*

Diverticulitis: No solid foods can be eaten at stage one, the clear liquids diet. Spelt is an excellent source of fiber.

Histamine: Low histamine. Check for gluten if avoiding gluten.

Lectins: Grains are high in lectins. Avoid.

Oxalates: Difficult to find reliable information. Test carefully.

Salicylates: Spelt is low in salicylates and while it's technically a type of wheat, this is an ancient form that many people on gluten-free diets can tolerate.

Spinach

- DASH: Fat: ✓ Sodium: ✓ Sugar: ✓
- Diverticulitis: Stage 1: ✗ Stage 2: 😕 Stage 3: ✓
- Histamine: ✗
- Lectin: ✓
- Oxalate: ✗
- Salicylates: 😕

DASH Diet (Hypertension): Spinach is an excellent vegetable to include on the DASH diet, containing vitamin K, potassium, and loads of antioxidants (source: *BBC Good Food*). Eat 4-5 servings of vegetables a day. *Saturated fat content: 0.06g (per 100g), Sodium content: 79 mg (per 100g), 3% daily value based on a 2,000 calorie diet, Sugar content: 0.4g (per 100g).*

Diverticulitis: No solid foods can be eaten at stage one, the clear liquids diet. Allowed on a high-fiber diet but test cautiously at the low-fiber stage.

Histamine: One of those foods generally considered 'healthy' but unfortunately high in histamine.

Lectins: Thought to be low-lectin.

Oxalates: Very high in oxalates. One of the highest oxalate foods. The website WebMD notes; *"Leafy greens like spinach contain many vitamins and minerals, but they're also high in oxalates. A half-cup of cooked spinach contains 755 milligrams."* If you must eat spinach, it's thought cooking it may reduce the oxalate levels, but only to around 650 mg per half cup.

Salicylates: Fresh spinach contains a moderately high level of salicylates. However, there is a hack that some people swear by. If you like spinach and want to enjoy its many beneficial nutrients with high amounts of carotenoids and a rich amount of vitamins A, C, K, iron, and potassium, try it frozen. Frozen spinach may be better tolerated on a low-salicylate diet but must be tested carefully.

Spirits

- DASH: Fat: ✓ Sodium: ✓ Sugar: ✓
- Diverticulitis: Stage 1: ✗ Stage 2: ✗ Stage 3: ✗
- Histamine: ✗
- Lectin: 😕
- Oxalate: ✓
- Salicylates: ✗

Spirits include brandy, gin, tequila, whiskey, vodka and flavored liquors (source: *The Spruce Eats*).

DASH Diet (Hypertension): *Drink alcohol sparingly on the DASH diet. You don't have to eliminate alcohol completely, although limiting consumption is good. Saturated fat content: 0g, Sodium content: 1mg, less than 1% daily value based on a 2,000 calorie diet, Sugar content: 0g.*

Diverticulitis: See "alcohol".

Histamine: Avoid. See "alcohol".

Lectins: As studies on spirits and lectins are limited, we recommend proceeding cautiously. See "alcohol" for more on spirits and lectins.

Oxalates: See alcohol.

Salicylates: Alcoholic beverages contain a high level of salicylates. See "alcohol" for more details.

Squashes

- DASH: Fat: ✓ Sodium: ✓ Sugar: ✓
- Diverticulitis: Stage 1: ✗ Stage 2: 😕 Stage 3: ✓
- Histamine: ✓
- Lectin: ✗
- Oxalate: 😕
- Salicylates: ✗

DASH Diet (Hypertension): *Allowed. Try spaghetti squash instead of pasta to reduce the calories.* **Butternut squash**: *Saturated fat content: 0g (per 100g), Sodium content: 4mg (per 100g), less than 1% daily value based on a 2,000 calorie diet, Sugar content: 2.2g (per 100g).* **Spaghetti squash**: *Saturated fat content: 0.1g (per 100g), Sodium content: 17mg (per 100g), less than 1% daily value based on a 2,000 calorie diet, Sugar content: 2.8g (per 100g).* **Summer squash**: *Saturated fat content: 0g (per 100g), Sodium content: 2mg (per 100g), less than 1% daily value based on a 2,000 calorie diet, Sugar content: 2.2g (per 100g).*

Diverticulitis: No solid foods can be eaten at stage one, the clear liquids diet. Allowed on the high-fiber diet. Peeling and deseeding help to reduce fiber content. Test carefully at the low-fiber stage.

Histamine: Tolerated.

Lectins: Thought to be high in lectin. Peeling and deseeding help to reduce lectin content.

Oxalates: Squash seeds are thought to be low, or low to moderate, 5-10mg per 100 grams. Cooked summer squash and winter squash are moderate, 10 - 25mg per 100 grams (source: *Urinary Stones - The Oxalate Content Of Food*).

Salicylates: Avoid. Thought to be high in salicylates.

Stevia

- DASH: Fat: ✓ Sodium: ✓ Sugar: ✓
- Diverticulitis: Stage 1: ✓ Stage 2: ✗ Stage 3: ✗
- Histamine: ✓
- Lectin: ✓
- Oxalate: 😕
- Salicylates: 😕

A processed sugar substitute, Stevia is made from a plant leaf and is in the Asteraceae family. Use it in coffee, tea, or baking instead of traditional sugar to reduce sugar consumption.

DASH Diet (Hypertension): Allowed. *Saturated fat content: 0g (per 100g), Sodium content: 0g (per 100g), less than 1% daily value based on a 2,000 calorie diet, Sugar content: 0g (per 100g).*

Diverticulitis: Sweeteners such as stevia may aggravate diverticulitis symptoms, so best to avoid them.

Histamine: Our favorite natural sweetener includes stevia leaves, liquid, and powder.

Lectins: Tolerated on a low-lectin diet.

Oxalates: Plenty of disagreement online about stevia (as there are many foods in this book). Website WebMD puts stevia in their high oxalate food category. Chemical stevia has no oxalate.

Salicylates: It does not appear to have been tested; however, most salicylate-sensitive people can tolerate them. Be cautious until you know how your body will react. It may not be the best choice if you have an allergy to ragweed.

Stinging nettle

- DASH: Fat: ✓ Sodium: ✓ Sugar: ✓
- Diverticulitis: Stage 1: 😕 Stage 2: ✗ Stage 3: ✓
- Histamine: ✗
- Lectin: ✗
- Oxalate: 😕
- Salicylates: 😕

Be sure to research the proper way to prepare stinging nettles before eating them, as they need to be cooked in order to become edible. But after that, stinging nettles are a healthy choice, chock full of vitamin A and vitamin C (source: *Eat Weeds*).

DASH Diet (Hypertension): *Saturated fat content: 0g (per 100g), Sodium content: 4 mg (per 100g) less than 1% daily value based on a 2,000 calorie diet, Sugar content: 0.3g (per 100g).*

Diverticulitis: No solid foods can be eaten at stage one, the clear liquids diet. Nettle tea with no milk or cream is allowed. Nettle is also allowed on the high-fiber diet.

Histamine: Alison Vickery quotes some excellent studies which suggest nettle is a potent antihistamine (working at the H1 receptor) and mast cell stabilizer. Approach cautiously as some still react to nettle tea.

Lectins: A study found "unusual" lectins in stinging nettles (source: *Science Direct: An unusual lectin from stinging nettle (Urtica dioica) rhizomes*). Best to avoid.

Oxalates: Stinging nettle can help prevent and possibly dissolve kidney stones and gout because its extract decreases elevated levels of calcium, oxalate, and creatinine in urine. One study showed it significantly limited the amount of calcium and oxalate and calcium oxalate crystals in the kidneys of test rats (source: *Pubmed*).

Salicylates: There is very little information on the amount of salicylates in stinging nettle. Some anecdotally report that it is likely to contain at least some salicylates, while others note it is free of the compound, making it impossible to rate accurately.

Strawberry

- DASH: Fat: ✓ Sodium: ✓ Sugar: ✓
- Diverticulitis: Stage 1: ✗ Stage 2: ✗ Stage 3: ✓

- Histamine: ✗
- Lectin: ✓
- Oxalate: ✓
- Salicylates: ✗

DASH Diet (Hypertension): Strawberries are full of vitamin C and ripe with health benefits. Some studies suggest strawberries may be helpful in a diet intended to reduce blood pressure. Researchers conducted a large study with over 34,000 people with hypertension. They found that those with the highest intake of anthocyanins — mainly from blueberries and strawberries — had an 8 percent reduction in the risk of high blood pressure, compared to those with a low anthocyanin intake (source: *Medical News Today*). *Saturated fat content: 0g (per 100g), Sodium content: 1 mg (per 100g), less than 1% daily value based on a 2,000 calorie diet, Sugar content: 4.9g (per 100g).*

Diverticulitis: No solid foods can be eaten at stage one, the clear liquids diet. Allowed on the high-fiber diet.

Histamine: High. Mast Cell 360 notes that strawberries may be tolerated in very small amounts (i.e. 1 strawberry).

Lectins: Contains relatively low lectins.

Oxalates: Thought to be low in oxalates. Winchester Hospital lists strawberries in their Foods safe-to-eat category.

Salicylates: Very high in salicylates.

Sugar

- DASH: Fat: ✓ Sodium: ✓ Sugar: ✗
- Diverticulitis: Stage 1: ✓ Stage 2: ✓ Stage 3: ✗
- Histamine: ✓
- Lectin: ✗
- Oxalate: ✓
- Salicylates: ✓

DASH Diet (Hypertension): Try to limit sugar intake. *Saturated fat content: 0g (per 100g), Sodium content: 1 mg (per 100g), less than 1% daily value based on a 2,000 calorie diet, Sugar content: 100g (per 100g).*

Diverticulitis: Sugar contains no fiber, so they're allowed on the low-fiber diet.

Histamine: Sugar may be low in histamine but is not good for those with health issues. With sugar, try natural alternatives. Stevia and monk fruit are the best natural alternatives. Inulin is another one to try.

Lectins: Avoid. While we realize that is easier said than done, sugar is not actually required in your diet and consuming too much can raise blood pressure (source: *Havard Health*). Opt for honey as an alternative to sugar - but still, use in moderation.

Oxalates: Sugar is thought to be low oxalate but is not good for those with certain health issues. Look into alternatives. The University of Chicago writes on its Kidney Stones site: *"Just one sugary drink raises your urine calcium within 30 minutes and keeps it up for at least 2 hours more. At the same time, it lowers your urine volume. If you have hypercalciuria - a majority of stone formers have it - the effect is larger because you start higher, and your urine volume will fall more. So with every sugary treat, the risk of making stones increases for hours."*

Salicylates: Standard white sugar is free of salicylates; however, it's believed to be a big contributor to the obesity epidemic and can increase the risk of developing many other health conditions. Lecture over.

Sunflower oil

- DASH: Fat: ✗ Sodium: ✓ Sugar: ✓
- Diverticulitis: Stage 1: ✗ Stage 2: ✓ Stage 3: ✗
- Histamine: 😐
- Lectin: ✗
- Oxalate: ✓
- Salicylates: ✗

DASH Diet (Hypertension): Sunflower oil is popular for cooking because of its high smoke point. However, it is high in saturated fats, so try to avoid them. *Saturated fat content: 13g (per 100g), Sodium content: 0mg (per 100g), less than 1% daily value based on a 2,000 calorie diet, Sugar content: 0g (per 100g).*

Diverticulitis: Sunflower oil contains no fiber, so they're allowed on the low-fiber diet.

Histamine: Medium histamine. We've noticed it can cause inflammation. This also goes for Rapeseed/Canola oil, but you might well find it agrees with you, and some sites note it is generally low histamine.

Lectins: High in lectins. One to put on your 'avoid' list.

Oxalates: Low oxalate, however, can cause inflammation. Test carefully.

Salicylates: Negligible amount of salicylates. There's a big but coming though. The website *Food Can Make You Ill* notes; "*Margarine and processed rapeseed (canola), safflower, soya bean, sunflower oils although low in salicylate are likely to contain preservatives that may mimic salicylate reactions and are best avoided.*"

Sunflower seeds

- DASH: Fat: ✗ Sodium: ✓ Sugar: ✓
- Diverticulitis: Stage 1: ✗ Stage 2: ✗ Stage 3: ✓
- Histamine: ✗
- Lectin: ✗
- Oxalate: ✓
- Salicylates: ✓

DASH Diet (Hypertension): Sunflower seeds are a great source of vitamin E, which protects the body from free radicals. *Saturated fat content: 4.5g (per 100g), Sodium content: 9 mg (per 100g) less than 1% daily value based on a 2,000 calorie diet, Sugar content: 2.6g (per 100g).*

Diverticulitis: No solid foods can be eaten at stage one, the clear liquids diet. Allowed on the high-fiber diet.

Histamine: High. We also notice sunflower seeds cause a general inflammation related to histamine, but this is anecdotal, and you may well have a different experience.

Lectins: High in lectins. To reduce lectin content, Precision Nutrition recommends soaking and cooking sunflower seeds. This is because the highest concentration of lectins can be found in the seeds of plants (source: *Diagnosis Diet*).

Oxalates: Low, just 3 mg oxalate per 1/4 cup (source: *https://www.thekidneydietitian.org/low-oxalate-nuts/*)

Salicylates: Very low amount of salicylates.

Sweetcorn

- DASH: Fat: ✓ Sodium: ✓ Sugar: ✓
- Diverticulitis: Stage 1: ✗ Stage 2: ✗ Stage 3: ✓
- Histamine: ✓

- Lectin: ✗
- Oxalate: 😖
- Salicylates: 😖

Also known as *corn on the cob*.

DASH Diet (Hypertension): Sweetcorn has a high fiber content, which may aid digestion and decrease the risk of heart disease (source: *Birds Eye*). Saturated fat content: 0.2g (per 100g), Sodium content: 15mg (per 100g), less than 1% daily value based on a 2,000 calorie diet, Sugar content: 3.2g (per 100g).

Diverticulitis: No solid foods can be eaten at stage one, the clear liquids diet. Allowed on the high-fiber diet.

Histamine: Tolerated.

Lectins: High in lectins. Corn is very resistant to heat; therefore, it's hard to reduce the lectin content.

Oxalates: Moderate.

Salicylates: Fresh sweetcorn is low in salicylates; however, canned sweetcorn may contain a moderate amount.

Sweet potato

- DASH: Fat: ✓ Sodium: ✓ Sugar: ✓
- Diverticulitis: Stage 1: ✗ Stage 2: ✓ Stage 3: ✓
- Histamine: ✓
- Lectin: ✓
- Oxalate: ✗
- Salicylates: ✗

Also known as *yams*.

DASH Diet (Hypertension): Sweet potatoes are rich in potassium, making them helpful for lowering blood pressure (source: *Medical News Today*). Saturated fat content: 0g (per 100g), Sodium content: 55 mg (per 100g), less than 1% daily value based on a 2,000 calorie diet, Sugar content: 4.2g (per 100g).

Diverticulitis: No solid foods can be eaten at stage one, the clear liquids diet. Peel the sweet potato on a low-fiber diet.

Histamine: Allowed.

Lectins: Unlike white potatoes, sweet potatoes are thought to be low in lectins and high in antioxidants. A much better source for your potato needs on a low-lectin diet.

Oxalates: Considered to be very high in oxalates, with some estimating 28 mg per 100 g (source: *Scientific Electronic Library Online of Brazil*). Dr. Jockers says this on his excellent website: "*I teach my clients to minimize their consumption of spinach, beets, grains, nuts, sweet potatoes and chocolate for 3 months.* "

Salicylates: Yellow sweet potatoes have a moderate amount of salicylates, and sweet potatoes are considered high in salicylates.

Tea, black

- DASH: Fat: ✓ Sodium: ✓ Sugar: ✓
- Diverticulitis: Stage 1: ✓ Stage 2: ✓ Stage 3: ✗
- Histamine: ✗
- Lectin: ✓

- Oxalate: ✗
- Salicylates: ✗

DASH Diet (Hypertension): Black tea is full of antioxidants that may boost heart health. Drink it hot or iced, and refrain from adding any extra sugar to it. *Saturated fat content: 0g (per 100g), Sodium content: 3 mg (per 100g), less than 1% daily value based on a 2,000 calorie diet, Sugar content: 0g (per 100g).*

Diverticulitis: Tea with no milk or cream is allowed at stage one, the clear liquid diet. Tea contains no fiber, so they're allowed on the low-fiber diet.

Histamine: The Histamine Intolerance Awareness Site lists black tea under *'foods that have been reported to block the diamine oxidase (DAO) enzyme'*.

Lectins: It's thought that tea is acceptable on a low-lectin diet.

Oxalates: Some teas, including black teas, are thought to accumulate a large amount of oxalates, resulting in a recommendation to eliminate black tea from your diet if you form oxalate stones (source: *nature.com*). In a 2003 study, researchers from New Zealand discovered a 'tea hack'. They noted;
"These studies show that consuming black tea on a daily basis will lead to a moderate intake of soluble oxalate each day, however the consumption of tea with milk regularly will cause the absorption of very little oxalate from tea."

Salicylates: Very high in salicylates.

Thyme

- DASH: Fat: ✓ Sodium: ✓ Sugar: ✓
- Diverticulitis: Stage 1: ✗ Stage 2: ✗ Stage 3: ✓
- Histamine: ✓
- Lectin: ✓
- Oxalate: ✓
- Salicylates: ✗

Thyme is a commonly used flavoring in meat, fish, and vegetable dishes.

DASH Diet (Hypertension): This herb has many healthy nutrients, such as potassium, vitamin A, and vitamin C (source: *WebMD*). *Saturated fat content: 0.5g (per 100g), Sodium content: 9 mg (per 100g), less than 1% daily value based on a 2,000 calorie diet, Sugar content: 0g (per 100g).*

Diverticulitis: Allowed on the high-fiber diet.

Histamine: Acceptable. Includes common thyme, German thyme, garden thyme

Lectins: Tolerated on a low-lectin diet.

Oxalates: Dried thyme is thought to contain low-to-moderate levels of oxalate.

Salicylates: Very high in salicylates.

Tomato

- DASH: Fat: ✓ Sodium: ✓ Sugar: ✓
- Diverticulitis: Stage 1: ✗ Stage 2: 😐 Stage 3: ✓
- Histamine: ✗
- Lectin: ✗
- Oxalate: ✗
- Salicylates: ✗

DASH Diet (Hypertension): Tomatoes are high in lycopene, which may reduce the risk of heart disease. Tomatoes can be consumed in many ways, from salads to sauces to sandwiches. *Saturated fat content: 0g (per 100g), Sodium content: 5mg (per 100g), less than 1% daily value based on a 2,000 calorie diet, Sugar content: 2.6g (per 100g).*

Diverticulitis: No solid foods can be eaten at stage one, the clear liquids diet. Peel, deseed and test cautiously on the low-fiber diet. Allowed at the high-fiber stage.

Histamine: High and includes tomato juice. On the Healing Histamine Site, author Yasmina notes how important it is to reintroduce 'healthy' higher histamine foods such as tomatoes once you start to feel better.

Lectins: High in lectins. One to put on your 'avoid' list. They're a part of the nightshade family, which is thought to be high in lectins, particularly in the seeds and peels. Precision Nutrition recommends something rather fiddly but potentially helpful. It suggests peeling and deseeding tomatoes before cooking to reduce the lectin content. This is because the highest concentration of lectins can be found in the seeds of plants (source: *Diagnosis Diet*).

Oxalates: Moderate to high.

Salicylates: Fresh tomato seems lower than canned tomatoes, tomato paste, and tomato sauce in terms of salicylates. And then there's a distinction between raw tomato and cooked tomato. The website Allergenics notes; *"Salicylates are found in plants, and in higher concentrations in plants that are concentrated by drying or juicing or making into sauces, pastes or jams. So while tomatoes may be high in salicylates, tomato paste will be higher. Raw tomatoes will have higher levels than cooked tomatoes though- it's tricky!"*

Trout

- DASH: Fat: ✗ Sodium: ✓ Sugar: ✓
- Diverticulitis: Stage 1: ✗ Stage 2: ✓ Stage 3: ✗
- Histamine: 😕
- Lectin: ✗
- Oxalate: ✓
- Salicylates: ✓

DASH Diet (Hypertension): Fish like trout are an excellent source of protein. Trout is low in mercury, making it a safe choice to include in a healthy diet (source: *SF Gate*). *Saturated fat content: 1.4g (per 100g), Sodium content: 51mg (per 100g), 2% daily value based on a 2,000 calorie diet, Sugar content: 0g (per 100g).*

Diverticulitis: No solid foods can be eaten at stage one, the clear liquids diet. Seafood contains no fiber, so trout is allowed on the low-fiber diet.

Histamine: Worth a comment as SIGHI notes freshwater brown trout, brook trout, and rainbow trout are low histamine. That's not our experience but may be for others.

Lectins: A study found lectins reported in trout (source: *Ng TB, Fai Cheung RC, Wing Ng CC, Fang EF, Wong JH. A review of fish lectins*), although we're unclear on the amount of lectins and whether these are harmful. Trout and salmon are closely related as they belong to the same fish family (source: *The Kitchen Community*). Salmon is acceptable on a low lectin diet, so maybe trout is too. Test carefully.

Oxalates: See fish.

Salicylates: Fish contains no to only trace amounts of salicylates, according to most reliable sources.

Tuna

- DASH: Fat: ✓ Sodium: ✓ Sugar: ✓
- Diverticulitis: Stage 1: ✗ Stage 2: ✓ Stage 3: ✗

- Histamine: ✗
- Lectin: ✓
- Oxalate: ✓
- Salicylates: ✓

DASH Diet (Hypertension): Tuna is high in protein and B vitamins (source: *BBC Good Food*). Canned tuna can be eaten conveniently, or cook fresh tuna with vegetables for a delicious meal. *Saturated fat content: 0.4g (per 100g), Sodium content: 47mg (per 100g), 1% daily value based on a 2,000 calorie diet, Sugar content: 0g (per 100g).*

Diverticulitis: No solid foods can be eaten at stage one, the clear liquids diet. Seafood contains no fiber, so tuna is allowed on the low-fiber diet.

Histamine: All canned food tends to be high in histamine. Tuna also tends to be high in heavy metals.

Lectins: Low in lectins. For a healthier option, opt for wild-caught tuna. These are thought to be less contaminated from man-made toxins as the fish feed on a natural diet (source: *The Nest*). Often thought to be high in mercury, so eat rarely.

Oxalates: Like most fish, it's low in oxalates, but tends to have a high heavy metal content.

Salicylates: Fish contains no to only trace amounts of salicylates, according to most reliable sources. Canned tuna often contains high mercury levels.

Turkey

- DASH: Fat: ✗ Sodium: ✓ Sugar: ✓
- Diverticulitis: Stage 1: ✗ Stage 2: ✓ Stage 3: ✗
- Histamine: ✓
- Lectin: ✓
- Oxalate: ✓
- Salicylates: ✓

DASH Diet (Hypertension): Turkey is lean meat and a good choice for the DASH diet. *Saturated fat content: 2.2g (per 100g), Sodium content: 103mg (per 100g), 4% daily value based on a 2,000 calorie diet, Sugar content: 0g (per 100g).*

Diverticulitis: No solid foods can be eaten at stage one, the clear liquids diet. Meat contains no fiber, so turkey is allowed on a low-fiber diet.

Histamine: Low histamine. See other comments about preferably eating organic and freshly cooked. No leftovers.

Lectins: Tolerated on a low-lectin diet. Opt for pasture-raised turkey.

Oxalates: Meat has little to no oxalates.

Salicylates: See "Meat"

Turmeric

- DASH: Fat: ✗ Sodium: ✓ Sugar: ✓
- Diverticulitis: Stage 1: ✗ Stage 2: ✗ Stage 3: ✓
- Histamine: ✓
- Lectin: ✓
- Oxalate: ✗
- Salicylates: ✗

DASH Diet (Hypertension): Turmeric is a spice rich in health benefits. It contains natural anti-inflammatory compounds and antioxidants. *Saturated fat content: 3.1g (per 100g), Sodium content: 38mg (per 100g), 1% daily value based on a 2,000 calorie diet, Sugar content: 3.2g (per 100g).*

Diverticulitis: Allowed on the high-fiber diet.

Histamine: Inflammation-fighting and low histamine.

Lectins: Packed with antioxidants and permitted on a low-lectin diet.

Oxalates: Sally K. Norton lists Turmeric as the highest oxalate-containing spice. She has an interesting suggestion for replacing turmeric in your food: *"To replace (whole root) turmeric use a turmeric extract sold as a dietary supplement. (Start with 1-3 caps per recipe, opened, and the capsule discarded.) (Oxalate sticks to fibers and other elements removed when an extract is made.)"*

Salicylates: Thought to be very high in salicylates.

Turnip

- DASH: Fat: ✔ Sodium: ✔ Sugar: ✔
- Diverticulitis: Stage 1: ✘ Stage 2: ✘ Stage 3: ✔
- Histamine: 😐
- Lectin: ✔
- Oxalate: ✘
- Salicylates: 😐

DASH Diet (Hypertension): Turnips contain dietary nitrates that may help to reduce blood pressure, making them a fantastic food to include in the DASH diet (source: *Medical News Today*). *Saturated fat content: 0g (per 100g), Sodium content: 67mg (per 100g), 2% daily value based on a 2,000 calorie diet, Sugar content: 3.8g (per 100g).*

Diverticulitis: No solid foods can be eaten at stage one, the clear liquids diet. Allowed on the high-fiber diet.

Histamine: Medium histamine and includes turnip greens, turnip roots and turnip cabbage.

Lectins: Falls under the cruciferous vegetable family (includes broccoli, kale, cabbage, radish etc.). These are considered low lectin and rich in vitamin C, folate and fiber.

Oxalates: Very high in oxalates, 30 mg per 100 g (source: *University of Chicago*).

Salicylates: Some conflicting information, categorized as low to moderate in salicylates depending on the source.

Vanilla

- DASH: Fat: ✔ Sodium: ✔ Sugar: ✘
- Diverticulitis: Stage 1: ✘ Stage 2: ✔ Stage 3: ✘
- Histamine: 😐
- Lectin: ✔
- Oxalate: ✘
- Salicylates: ✘

Includes vanilla, vanilla extract, vanilla pod, vanilla powder, and vanilla sugar. Vanilla is often used as a flavoring in baked goods and desserts. It can be used as a substitute for sugar to add some sweetness to foods.

DASH Diet (Hypertension): Allowed. *Saturated fat content: 0g (per 100g), Sodium content: 9mg (per 100g), less than 1% daily value based on a 2,000 calorie diet, Sugar content: 13g (per 100g).*

Diverticulitis: No solid foods can be eaten at stage one, the clear liquids diet. Vanilla contains no fiber, so they're allowed on the low-fiber diet.

Histamine: Medium histamine. Please note - vanilla essence is often in alcohol, so it tends to be a poorer choice.

Lectins: Allowed on a low-lectin diet.

Oxalates: Lists vary. Challenging to get consistent information and therefore avoid.

Salicylates: Avoid.

Venison

- DASH: Fat: ✗ Sodium: ✓ Sugar: ✓
- Diverticulitis: Stage 1: ✗ Stage 2: ✓ Stage 3: ✗
- Histamine: ✓
- Lectin: ✓
- Oxalate: ✓
- Salicylates: ✓

Meat from the deer. Venison has more protein than any other red meat. It is also rich in iron.

DASH Diet (Hypertension): Red meat should be limited or avoided in the DASH diet. *Saturated fat content: 1.3g (per 100g), Sodium content: 54mg (per 100g), 2% daily value based on a 2,000 calorie diet, Sugar content: 0g (per 100g).*

Diverticulitis: No solid foods can be eaten at stage one, the clear liquids diet. Meat contains no fiber, so venison is allowed on the low-fiber diet.

Histamine: Tolerated.

Lectins: Tolerated. Opt for grass-fed venison.

Oxalates: See "Meat"

Salicylates: See "Meat"

Vinegar: balsamic

- DASH: Fat: ✓ Sodium: ✓ Sugar: ✗
- Diverticulitis: Stage 1: ✗ Stage 2: ✓ Stage 3: ✗
- Histamine: ✗
- Lectin: ✓
- Oxalate: ✓
- Salicylates: ✗

DASH Diet (Hypertension): Some studies have suggested that balsamic vinegar can help to reduce cholesterol levels (source: *Healthline*). *Saturated fat content: 0g (per 100g), Sodium content: 23 mg (per 100g), less than 1% daily value based on a 2,000 calorie diet, Sugar content: 15g (per 100g).*

Diverticulitis: Contains no fiber, so they're allowed on the low-fiber diet.

Histamine: Avoid.

Lectins: It's thought that all types of vinegar are permitted on a low-lectin diet.

Oxalates: 5-10 mg per 100 g, low (source: *Urinary Stones - The Oxalate Content Of Food*).

Salicylates: We believe them to be moderate to high in salicylates. However, LiveStrong notes; *"Fennel, vinegar and soy sauce contain moderate amounts"*.

Vinegar: distilled white vinegar

- DASH: Fat: ✓ Sodium: ✓ Sugar: ✓
- Diverticulitis: Stage 1: ✗ Stage 2: ✓ Stage 3: ✗
- Histamine: ✗
- Lectin: ✓
- Oxalate: ✓
- Salicylates: ✗

DASH Diet (Hypertension): Some studies suggest that consuming white vinegar may reduce blood sugar levels after meals (source: *Healthline*). Saturated fat content: 0g (per 100g), Sodium content: 2mg (per 100g), less than 1% daily value based on a 2,000 calorie diet, Sugar content: 0.04g (per 100g).

Diverticulitis: Contains no fiber, so they're allowed on the low-fiber diet.

Histamine: Avoid.

Lectins: It's thought that all types of vinegar are permitted on a low-lectin diet.

Oxalates: Very low, less than 5 mg per 100 g (source: *Urinary Stones - The Oxalate Content Of Food*).

Salicylates: High in salicylates. The website Allergenics notes; *"Sauces and Condiments: most commercial or store-bought gravies, sauces and pastes (eg. tomato paste, Worcester sauce, gravy mix), jams, marmalades, fruit/mint/honey flavoring, chewing gum, white and cider vinegars."* However, LiveStrong notes; *"Fennel, vinegar and soy sauce contain moderate amounts"*

Walnut

- DASH: Fat: ✗ Sodium: ✓ Sugar: ✓
- Diverticulitis: Stage 1: ✗ Stage 2: ✗ Stage 3: ✓
- Histamine: ✗
- Lectin: 🤔
- Oxalate: ✗
- Salicylates: 🤔

DASH Diet (Hypertension): Eating nuts such as walnuts may help to lower blood pressure (source: *Healthline*). Choose walnuts as a healthy midday snack. Saturated fat content: 6g (per 100g), Sodium content: 2mg (per 100g) less than 1% daily value based on a 2,000 calorie diet, Sugar content: 2.6g (per 100g).

Diverticulitis: No solid foods can be eaten at stage one, the clear liquids diet. Allowed on the high-fiber diet.

Histamine: Avoid.

Lectins: Mixed opinion. Some sources point to walnuts being acceptable on a low-lectin diet, whereas another source noted walnuts contain lectins. Test carefully.

Oxalates: Thought to be very high in oxalates. Some say all nuts should be avoided on a Low-Oxalate diet.

Salicylates: There is a bit of a debate about the amount of salicylates in walnuts, with some analyses showing high levels of salicylates and other reliable sources listing them as "moderate" in salicylates. Whether high or moderate, it seems walnut contains levels of salicylates that require a cautious approach.

Watercress

- DASH: Fat: ✓ Sodium: ✓ Sugar: ✓
- Diverticulitis: Stage 1: ✗ Stage 2: ✗ Stage 3: ✓

- Histamine: ✓
- Lectin: ✓
- Oxalate: ✗
- Salicylates: ✗

DASH Diet (Hypertension): Watercress contains nitrates that can help to lower blood pressure (source: *Watercress*). Add it to your salad for a healthy boost. *Saturated fat content: 0g (per 100g), Sodium content: 41mg (per 100g), 1% daily value based on a 2,000 calorie diet, Sugar content: 0.2g (per 100g).*

Diverticulitis: No solid foods can be eaten at stage one, the clear liquids diet. Allowed on the high-fiber diet.

Histamine: Potentially histamine-lowering. Alison Vickery notes a study which showed that the peppery-flavored watercress inhibits 60% of all histamine released from mast cells.

Lectins: Falls under the cruciferous vegetable family (includes broccoli, kale, cabbage, radish etc.). These are considered low-lectin and rich in vitamin C, folate and fiber.

Oxalates: High, best avoided. See cress for more info.

Salicylates: Watercress has a fairly high amount of salicylates.

Watermelon

- DASH: Fat: ✓ Sodium: ✓ Sugar: ✗
- Diverticulitis: Stage 1: ✗ Stage 2: ✓ Stage 3: ✗
- Histamine: 😐
- Lectin: ✗
- Oxalate: ✓
- Salicylates: 😐

DASH Diet (Hypertension): Watermelon is rich in three nutrients that can help reduce blood pressure—L-citrulline, lycopene, and potassium (source: *Eating Well*). *Saturated fat content: 0g (per 100g), Sodium content: 1mg (per 100g), less than 1% daily value based on a 2,000 calorie diet, Sugar content: 6g (per 100g).*

Diverticulitis: No solid foods can be eaten at stage one, the clear liquids diet. Low in fiber, so allowed on the low-fiber diet.

Histamine: The Histamine Intolerance Site lists melon as low histamine but please note, watermelon is listed in a different category as medium histamine and should be approached with real caution. Many people do not agree with watermelon when considering histamine. Fact vs Fitness puts watermelon on their 'allowed' list, so it's something you may want to approach with caution.

Lectins: Thought to contain high amounts of lectins.

Oxalates: See melon.

Salicylates: Watermelon was analyzed to contain moderate amounts of salicylates, while other melons, such as cantaloupe (also known as rock-melon), were shown to have a much higher level. There is some debate over watermelon, so approach cautiously. As it is such a close call, there is an inconsistency in site ratings, listed as either moderate or high depending on the source.

Wheat

- DASH: Fat: ✓ Sodium: ✓ Sugar: ✓
- Diverticulitis: Stage 1: ✗ Stage 2: 😐 Stage 3: 😐

- Histamine: 😖
- Lectin: ✗
- Oxalate: 😖
- Salicylates: ✓

DASH Diet (Hypertension): The DASH diet includes several servings of whole grains per day. Try to choose whole grains, which are rich in fiber and other nutrients (source: *Qardio*). *Saturated fat content: 0.2g (per 100g), Sodium content: 2mg (per 100g), less than 1% daily value based on a 2,000 calorie diet, Sugar content: 0.3g (per 100g).*

Diverticulitis: No solid foods can be eaten at stage one, the clear liquids diet. Fiber levels depend on the type of wheat. Whole wheat is thought to be high in fiber whereas refined wheat is thought to be low in fiber (source: *Healthline*).

Histamine: Medium histamine, and many people observe giving up gluten helps their overall histamine and wellness levels, so this is something to consider.

Lectins: Wheat is considered a grain of the seed (source: *Diagnosis Diet*). Grains are considered high in lectins and should be avoided. Look for gluten-free alternatives and check ingredients.

Oxalates: Some debate. Dr. Jockers lists in his High-Oxalate Food List category.

Salicylates: The grain of wheat is free of salicylates; however, as it's not eaten on its own when made into bread, you'll need to consider the other ingredients.

Wheat germ

- DASH: Fat: ✗ Sodium: ✓ Sugar: ✓
- Diverticulitis: Stage 1: ✗ Stage 2: ✗ Stage 3: ✓
- Histamine: ✗
- Lectin: ✗
- Oxalate: ✗
- Salicylates: ✓

The germ of cereal and part of a wheat kernel.

DASH Diet (Hypertension): Wheat germ can be added to foods to increase nutritional value. High in fiber, wheat germ is packed with healthy nutrients. Try it on top of oatmeal or yogurt, add it to a smoothie, or bake it into bread (source: *Bob's Red Mill*). *Saturated fat content: 1.7g (per 100g), Sodium content: 6mg (per 100g) less than 1% daily value based on a 2,000 calorie diet, Sugar content: 0g (per 100g).*

Diverticulitis: No solid foods can be eaten at stage one, the clear liquids diet. Allowed on the high-fiber diet.

Histamine: Avoid.

Lectins: As wheat is considered a grain of seed, we know grains are high in lectins. Avoid.

Oxalates: A study in Pubmed showed high total oxalate content (>50 mg/100 g) in the whole grain wheat species Triticum durum (76.6 mg/100 g), Triticum sativum (71.2 mg/100 g), and Triticum aestivum (53.3 mg/100 g).

Salicylates: Part of a wheat kernel that helps the plant reproduce, wheat germ is free of salicylate. Refer to "Wheat" for more details.

White button mushroom

- DASH: Fat: ✓ Sodium: ✓ Sugar: ✓
- Diverticulitis: Stage 1: ✗ Stage 2: 😖 Stage 3: ✓

- Histamine: 😕
- Lectin: ✓
- Oxalate: ✓
- Salicylates: ✓

White button mushrooms are the most popular mushroom variety (source: *Mushroom Council*).

DASH Diet (Hypertension): Allowed. Mushrooms can be prepared in many ways and eaten with a wide variety of dishes, so they're easy to include in your diet. Try them sautéed with pasta or on top of pizza. *Saturated fat content: 0.1g (per 100g), Sodium content: 5mg (per 100g) less than 1% daily value based on a 2,000 calorie diet, Sugar content: 2g (per 100g).*

Diverticulitis: No solid foods can be eaten at stage one, the clear liquids diet. Whilst mushroom doesn't contain the highest amounts of fiber compared to other veg. They can still be eaten on a high-fiber diet. Test carefully on a low-fiber diet.

Histamine: See "Mushrooms"

Lectins: Mushrooms fall under the lowest lectin content options for a low-lectin diet.

Oxalates: See "Mushrooms"

Salicylates: See "Mushrooms"

Wild rice

- DASH: Fat: ✓ Sodium: ✓ Sugar: ✓
- Diverticulitis: Stage 1: ✗ Stage 2: ✗ Stage 3: ✓
- Histamine: ✓
- Lectin: ✗
- Oxalate: 😕
- Salicylates: ✓

Not actually a rice - it's an aquatic grass (fun fact).

DASH Diet (Hypertension): A powerful source of antioxidants and may be a heart-healthy food to include in your diet. *Saturated fat content: 0.2g (per 100g), Sodium content: 7mg (per 100g), less than 1% daily value based on a 2,000 calorie diet, Sugar content: 2.5g (per 100g).*

Diverticulitis: No solid foods can be eaten at stage one, the clear liquids diet. Allowed on the high-fiber diet.

Histamine: See more comments on "Rice".

Lectins: Wild rice must be cooked longer than white and brown rice (source: *The Spruce Eats*). It's thought that using a pressure cooker and boiling rice reduces lectin content. Test carefully.

Oxalates: See comments on 'Rice'. Rice varies considerably by type.

Salicylates: Generally fine. See "Rice"

Wine

- DASH: Fat: ✓ Sodium: ✓ Sugar: ✓
- Diverticulitis: Stage 1: ✗ Stage 2: ✗ Stage 3: ✗
- Histamine: ✗
- Lectin: 😕

- Oxalate: ✓
- Salicylates: ✗

DASH Diet (Hypertension): Drink alcohol sparingly on the DASH diet. You don't have to eliminate alcohol completely, although limiting consumption is good. A study found molecules in red wine may cause a drop in blood pressure (source: *British Heart Foundation*). Many sources suggest red wine is high in antioxidants however, Dr. Robert Kloner, Chief Science Officer and Director of Cardiovascular Research at Huntington Medical Research Institutes, argues the amount you need to drink for protective effects is debatable as this would mean drinking too much wine. *Saturated fat content: 0g, Sodium content: 5mg (per 100g), less than 1% daily value based on a 2,000 calorie diet, Sugar content: 0.8g.*

Diverticulitis: See alcohol.

Histamine: Alcohols are some of the most problematic things you can consume on a low histamine diet. Wines are often extremely difficult, although some low-histamine wines can be found. But note the DAO-blocking element in the 'Alcohol' section. Alcohols contain histamine-degrading enzymes, but some rums, tequilas and Tito's Vodka may be purer than others. We have seen some claims online that plain vodka, gin and white rum are all low in histamine - these may be better options than other alcohols, but they still may block your DAO enzyme and therefore cause a histamine reaction.

Lectins: It seems that dessert wines, sweet wines and white wines should be avoided. Given the high sugar content, these wines don't seem to have the same benefits as red wine. Red wine contains high levels of Polyphenols (antioxidants) compared to other types of wine (including white wine). Some experts permit drinking wine high in Polyphenols (in moderation) on a low-lectin diet. Note that the nutrition content of red wine depends on how the grapes are grown. For example, it's thought that grapes grown at a higher altitude have greater exposure to the sun. Hence, they contain higher levels of Polyphenols (source: *Katherine Senko: Polyphenols in Wine*).

Oxalates: See alcohol.

Salicylates: Alcoholic beverages tend to contain a high level of salicylates. See "alcohol" for more details.

Yam

- DASH: Fat: ✓ Sodium: ✓ Sugar: ✓
- Diverticulitis: Stage 1: ✗ Stage 2: ✗ Stage 3: ✓
- Histamine: ✓
- Lectin: ✓
- Oxalate: ✗
- Salicylates: 🤐

Also known as *sweet potatoes*.

DASH Diet (Hypertension): Allowed. Yams are a great source of fiber and vitamin C (source: *Fruits and Veggies*). *Saturated fat content: 0g (per 100g), Sodium content: 9mg (per 100g), less than 1% daily value based on a 2,000 calorie diet, Sugar content: 0.5g (per 100g).*

Diverticulitis: No solid foods can be eaten at stage one, the clear liquids diet. Allowed on the high-fiber diet.

Histamine: Tolerated.

Lectins: Tolerated.

Oxalates: Very high in oxalates, 40 mg per 100 g (source: *University of Chicago*).

Salicylates: See "Potatoes"

Yeast

- DASH: Fat: ✔ Sodium: ✔ Sugar: ✔
- Diverticulitis: Stage 1: ✘ Stage 2: ✘ Stage 3: ✔
- Histamine: 😐
- Lectin: ✘
- Oxalate: ✘
- Salicylates: ✘

Often used in baking, particularly bread.

DASH Diet (Hypertension): Allowed. *Saturated fat content: 0.6g (per 100g), Sodium content: 50mg (per 100g), 2% daily value based on a 2,000 calorie diet, Sugar content: 0g (per 100g).*

Diverticulitis: No solid foods can be eaten at stage one, the clear liquids diet. Allowed on the high-fiber diet.

Histamine: Varies from batch to batch. Applies to fresh and dried, approach with extreme caution.

Lectins: One to put on your 'avoid' list.

Oxalates: Yeast as a baking ingredient has been found moderately high in oxalate content.

Salicylates: Salicylates are present in yeast extracts (source: *Australian Allergy Centre*). Avoid.

Yogurt/Yoghurt

- DASH: Fat: ✔ Sodium: ✔ Sugar: ✔
- Diverticulitis: Stage 1: ✘ Stage 2: ✔ Stage 3: ✘
- Histamine: ✘
- Lectin: 😐
- Oxalate: ✔
- Salicylates: ✔

Produced by fermenting milk and bacteria.

DASH Diet (Hypertension): Low or non-fat yogurt can be a great choice to add to your diet. Enjoy it for breakfast or a snack, paired with fresh berries. *Saturated fat content: 0.1g (per 100g), Sodium content: 36mg (per 100g), 1% daily value based on a 2,000 calorie diet, Sugar content: 3.2g (per 100g).*

Diverticulitis: Avoid at stage one the clear liquid diet as yogurt is made of milk which causes flare-ups. All liquids should be clear. Yogurt contains no fiber, so they're allowed on a low-fiber diet.

Histamine: Unfortunately, almost always high histamine. You could try making your own batch with low histamine bacteria.

Lectins: A study found the fermentation process reduces lower lectin content (source: *Sá AGA, Moreno YMF, Carciofi BAM. Food processing for the improvement of plant proteins digestibility*). Be cautious of yogurt made from A1 casein protein and sweetened yogurt. Goat and sheep yogurt are acceptable on a low-lectin diet. Coconut yogurt may also be a suitable alternative, but please check other ingredients.

Oxalates: Very low in oxalate, although often high in sugar. The University of Virginia Digestive Health Center advises: *"Eat plenty of calcium-rich foods. Calcium binds to oxalate so that it isn't absorbed into your blood and cannot reach your kidneys. Dairy is free of oxalate and high in calcium, so it is an ideal choice. Choose skim, low fat, or full-fat versions depending on your weight goals. If you are lactose intolerant, look for lactose-free dairy such as Lactaid brand, or eat yogurt or kefir instead."*

Salicylates: Yogurt is a calcium-rich food that is free of salicylates. However, for optimal health, avoid versions with sugars and additives, ideally choosing plain yogurt mixed with a low-salicylate fruit or nuts for added flavor and crunch.

Zucchini

- DASH: Fat: ✓ Sodium: ✓ Sugar: ✓
- Diverticulitis: Stage 1: ✗ Stage 2: ✗ Stage 3: ✓
- Histamine: ✓
- Lectin: ✗
- Oxalate: ✓
- Salicylates: ✗

Also known as *courgette*.

DASH Diet (Hypertension): Rich in antioxidants and may promote heart health. Include zucchini as part of a well-rounded diet. *Saturated fat content: 0.1g (per 100g), Sodium content: 8mg (per 100g), less than 1% daily value based on a 2,000 calorie diet, Sugar content: 2.5g (per 100g).*

Diverticulitis: No solid foods can be eaten at stage one, the clear liquids diet. Allowed on the high-fiber diet.

Histamine: Tolerated.

Lectins: There is mixed opinion on zucchini, but it is generally thought to be high in lectin content. Peeling and deseeding help to reduce lectin content, and some sources say it's ok to consume courgette/zucchini. Test carefully.

Oxalates: Thought to be low oxalate by most of our sources.

Salicylates: High in salicylates. It is often listed as the highest salicylate content in vegetables, alongside chicory, endive, and peppers.

SOURCES

These excellent sources come highly recommended in your further research on the various diets. As far as possible we have consulted all these sites in our research into this food list.

Please click on these top diet sites for further reading. We consider them to be the best sources out there.

DASH (Hypertension)

- Mayo Clinic - DASH diet: healthy eating to lower your blood pressure https://www.mayoclinic.org/healthy-lifestyle/nutrition-and-healthy-eating/in-depth/dash-diet/art-20048456#:~:text=The%20DASH%20diet%20is%20rich,and%20full%2Dfat%20dairy%20products.
- National Heart, Lung and Blood Institute (NIH) - DASH eating plan: https://www.nhlbi.nih.gov/education/dash-eating-plan
- Pub Med - Effects of blood pressure of reduced dietary sodium and the Dietary Approaches to Stop Hypertension (DASH) diet. DASH-Sodium Collaborative Research Group https://pubmed.ncbi.nlm.nih.gov/11136953/
- Trifecta Nutrition - DASH Diet (Hypertension) Guidelines and Food Lists https://www.trifectanutrition.com/health/dash-diet-guidelines-and-food-lists
- National Heart, Lung and Blood Institute (NIH) - Your guide to lowering your blood pressure with DASH - https://www.nhlbi.nih.gov/files/docs/public/heart/new_dash.pdf
- FDA - Sodium in your diet - https://www.fda.gov/food/nutrition-education-resources-materials/sodium-your-diet
- NHS - Sugar: the facts - https://www.nhs.uk/live-well/eat-well/how-does-sugar-in-our-diet-affect-our-health/
- Cleveland Clinic - Sodium controlled diet - https://my.clevelandclinic.org/health/articles/15426-sodium-controlled-diet

Diverticulitis:

- Dr Axe Diverticulitis Diet https://draxe.com/health/diverticulitis-diet/
- Cleveland Clinic - What's the Difference Between Soluble and Insoluble Fiber? https://health.clevelandclinic.org/whats-the-difference-between-soluble-and-insoluble-fiber/
- National Library of Medicine - Diverticular disease and diverticulitis: Surgery for diverticulitis and diverticular disease https://www.ncbi.nlm.nih.gov/books/NBK506997/
- Harvard Health Publishing - Harvard researchers link diverticulitis to red meat https://www.health.harvard.edu/digestive-health/harvard-researchers-link-diverticulitis-to-red-meat#:~:text=Now%2C%20a%20study%20published%20online,constipation%2C%20and%20even%20rectal%20bleeding.
- Medical News Today - Soluble and insoluble fiber: What is the difference https://www.medicalnewstoday.com/articles/319176#what-are-the-benefits-of-fiber
- University of Wisconsin-Madison - Study reveals gene expression changes with meditation https://news.wisc.edu/study-reveals-gene-expression-changes-with-meditation/

Histamine:

- Histamine Intolerance Awareness Site Food List - https://www.histamineintolerance.org.uk/about/the-food-diary/the-food-list/
- Alison Vickery Anti-Food List - https://www.alisonvickery.com/blog/anti-histamine-foods
- SFGATE Histamine Reducing Foods - https://healthyeating.sfgate.com/histaminereducing-foods-12197.html
- Factvsfitness Master List Of Low Histamine Foods - https://factvsfitness.com/blogs/news/histamine-intolerance-food-list
- SIGHI Food List - https://www.mastzellaktivierung.info/downloads/foodlist/21_FoodList_EN_alphabetic_withCateg.pdf
- The Histamine Intolerance Site Food List (referenced throughout with permission) https://histamineintolerance.net/foodlist
- MastCell360 Low and High Histamine Food Lists https://mastcell360.com/low-histamine-foods-list/
- Healing Histamine, Histamine In Food Lists https://healinghistamine.com/what-is-histamine/histamine-in-food-lists/

Lectins:

- Harvard T.H. Chan School of Public Health - Lectins https://www.hsph.harvard.edu/nutritionsource/anti-nutrients/lectins/
- Precision Nutrition - All about lectins https://www.precisionnutrition.com/all-about-lectins
- Dietetically Speaking - The lectin-free diet https://dieteticallyspeaking.com/the-lectin-free-diet/
- Mental Food Chain - 400+ foods high in lectins and lectin-free food list https://www.mentalfoodchain.com/foods-high-in-lectins/
- Amos Institute - What are lectins and the lectin-free diet? https://amosinstitute.com/blog/what-are-lectins-and-the-lectin-free-diet/
- Mayo Clinic - What are dietary lectins and should you avoid eating them? https://amosinstitute.com/blog/what-are-lectins-and-the-lectin-free-diet/
- Everyday Health - Lectin-Free Diet: Benefits, Risks, Food Choices, and More https://www.everydayhealth.com/diet-nutrition/lectin-free-diet/
- Dr. Steven Gundry Diet Food List https://gundrymd.com/dr-gundry-diet-food-list/
- Restart Med - Food List https://www.restartmed.com/wp-content/uploads/2018/09/Foods-high-in-Lectins-1.pdf
- Pritikin Longevitiy Center + Spa - Are nightshade vegetables bad for you? https://www.pritikin.com/are-nightshade-vegetables-bad
- Shawn Wells - Your guide to lectins, phytates & oxalates https://shawnwells.com/2020/07/your-guide-to-lectins-phytates-oxalates/
- Daytona Wellness Center - What should you eat https://daytonawellnesscenter.com/what-should-you-eat-published-june-18-2017-by-dr-daniel-thomas-do-ms/
- Healthline - Everything you need to know about dietary lectins https://www.healthline.com/nutrition/dietary-lectins
- Eating Well - What is the lectin-free diet? https://www.eatingwell.com/article/7827647/what-is-the-lectin-free-diet/
- Mind Body Green - Foods high in lectins: what to avoid to heal your gut https://www.mindbodygreen.com/articles/foods-high-in-lectins

Oxalates:

- The University of Chicago - How To Eat A Low Oxalate Diet https://kidneystones.uchicago.edu/how-to-eat-a-low-oxalate-diet/

Sources

- Harvard T.H. Chan School of Public Health https://regepi.bwh.harvard.edu/health/Oxalate/files
- Harvard T.H. Chan School of Public Health Food List https://regepi.bwh.harvard.edu/health/Oxalate/files/Oxalate%20Content%20of%20Foods.xls
- National Library of Medicine - Oxalate content of food: a tangled web https://pubmed.ncbi.nlm.nih.gov/25168533/
- University of Virginia - Digestive Health Center https://med.virginia.edu/ginutrition/wp-content/uploads/sites/199/2014/04/Oxalate-Foods-02.17.pdf
- Pitchaporn Wanyo, Kannika Huaisan & Tossaporn Chamsai - Oxalate contents of Thai rice paddy herbs (L. aromatica and L. geoffrayi) are affected by drying method and changes after cooking https://link.springer.com/article/10.1007/s42452-020-2703-6
- Urinary Stones Info - The Oxalate Content Of Food https://www.urinarystones.info/resources/Docs/Oxalate-content-of-food-2008.pdf
- Sally K. Norton Which Spices Are High In Oxalate https://sallyknorton.com/which-spices-are-high-in-oxalate/
- Low Oxalate Info Website http://lowoxalateinfo.com/
- Winchester Hospital Low-Oxalate Diet Health Library https://www.winchesterhospital.org/health-library/article?id=196214
- Low-Oxalate Diet - Mark O'Brien MD (adapted from University of Pittsburgh Medical Center https://www.markobrienmd.com/OxalateDiet.pdf
- University of Michigan Health - Foods High in Oxalate https://www.uofmhealth.org/health-library/aa166321

Salicylates:

- ResearchGate - A systematic review of salicylates in foods: Estimated daily intake of a Scottish population https://www.researchgate.net/publication/50197171_A_systematic_review_of_salicylates_in_foods_Estimated_daily_intake_of_a_Scottish_population
- Diet vs Disease – Salicylate Intolerance: The Complete Guide + List of Foods
- https://www.dietvsdisease.org/salicylate-intolerance/
- Journal of the American Dietetic Association – Salicylates in foods https://www.slhd.nsw.gov.au/rpa/allergy/research/salicylatesinfoods.pdf
- Food & Function – Natural salicylates: foods, functions and disease prevention
- https://pubmed.ncbi.nlm.nih.gov/21879102/
- Dr. Richard Coleman, Millhouse Integrative Medical Centre – MMC Fact Sheet 908 Salicylate Content of Foods http://www.millhousemedical.co.nz/files/docs/factsheet_8_salicylates_in_foods.pdf
- Journal of the American Dietetic Association - Are there foods that should be avoided if a patient is sensitive to salicylates? https://pubmed.ncbi.nlm.nih.gov/20497789/
- Nutrients journal – Effectiveness of Personalized Low Salicylate Diet in the Management of Salicylates Hypersensitive Patients: Interventional Study https://www.ncbi.nlm.nih.gov/pmc/articles/PMC8003553/
- Healthline – Salicylate Sensitivity: Causes, Symptoms and Foods to Avoid https://www.healthline.com/nutrition/salicylate-sensitivity
- Healthline – Should You Avoid Salicylates? https://www.healthline.com/nutrition/salicylate-sensitivity#TOC_TITLE_HDR_7
- Food Can Make You Ill Food List - https://www.foodcanmakeyouill.co.uk/salicylate-in-food.html
- WebMD – High Salicylate Foods - https://www.webmd.com/diet/high-salicylate-foods#1

Made in the USA
Middletown, DE
25 September 2022